Coronavirus-The Inside Story: Multidimensional Prevention and Treatment

Tom Garz

Published by TG Ideas LLC, 2020.

While every precaution has been taken in the preparation of this book, the publisher assumes no responsibility for errors or omissions, or for damages resulting from the use of the information contained herein.

CORONAVIRUS-THE INSIDE STORY:
MULTIDIMENSIONAL PREVENTION AND TREATMENT

First edition. June 25, 2020.

Copyright © 2020 Tom Garz.

ISBN: 978-1393807049

Written by Tom Garz.

Disclaimers

Use of the Information in this book may help the Patient, Doctor, and/or Others "Get Better".

Some common Side Effects may include:

- A better understanding of what affects Health and Symptoms,
- Seeing the big picture surrounding Symptoms,
- Better health, less dependence on medication/treatment, generally "feeling better",
- Experiencing less perceived stress, more contentment with self and life,
- Perceiving more control of your life, in general, realizing there are always options no matter what,
- New insights on what could be done to make "it" better.

Note - Continued Use of the Information in this book may result in "Staying Better".

Ask your Doctor if "Getting Better" and "Staying Better" are right for you. ☺

****

Seriously though....

This book is for information only and is not advice of any kind, especially not Medical and/or Legal Advice. The author of this book is a Non-Professional. Seek professional advice, as needed. This book is meant to help, but using this information is at your own risk. The author of this book has made efforts to make sure the referenced information is/was correct when the book was published. Efforts were also made to avoid plagiarism in this book by the writer. Any reference to any specific product or service is for information or example only and does not constitute or imply any endorsement, recommendation, or favoring by TG Ideas LLC. TG Ideas LLC does not assume any liability to anyone and hereby disclaims any loss, damage, disruption from any errors, omissions, perceived or actual unintentional plagiarism, whether such are caused by negligence, accident, or any other means. Additional Disclaimers are at https://sites.google.com/site/tgideas/ideas-for-products-or-services/disclaimer

Summary - I'm not a Healthcare Professional. I wrote this book based on my personal learnings/experience and the References at the end of this Book. This book is for your information only and is not medical advice.

****

How to Use This or Most any E-Book

Did you know you could use e-books in many ways, other than just reading from an e-book reader?

- Yes, you can read my e-book on most any e-book reader. I hope you like it and find it helpful.
- You can print out a copy to use alongside my e-book, though the printout won't have the hyperlinks that are in my e-book. In addition, the print layout might not look the same, but it might suit your purposes.
- You could manage my e-book for your purposes with the open-source tool, Calibre[1].
- You can add your own personal notes and highlighting to my e-book, for your use, depending on which e-book reader you are using.
- The hyperlinks were known to work at the time of publication. Due to the ever-changing environment of the Internet, the links might not work in the future. If this happens, simply copy the text and put quotes around the copied text, then do an Internet search. The quotes tell the search engine to look for an exact match. For example, if the link for Pulse diagnosis[2] doesn't work someday, then do an Internet search for **"Pulse diagnosis"**. What you're looking for will probably be near the top of the Internet Search Results.
- The Chapter References provided in this book are by no means a complete listing. Only a few references are provided for each chapter to illustrate the concept within the text. If a particular reference is of interest to you, then just search for

---

1. https://calibre-ebook.com/

2. https://en.wikipedia.org/wiki/Pulse_diagnosis

the title of the reference. By doing so, you will "find more like this".

- Furthermore, in most of my books, Internet Search Strings are provided for your use. If provided, use these strings as a start for you to "find more like this". Of course, you could modify the strings to find exactly what you're looking for.

References –

6 Android Ebook Reader Apps With Great Annotation Features[3]

Beyond Highlighting: How to Get the Most From Your Annotations[4]

The Simple Guide to Annotations: How to Annotate PDFs, Ebooks, Images, and Websites[5]

Annotating & Highlighting E-Books[6]

How to Print, E-mail or Save EBSCO eBooks Pages as a PDF[7]

Calibre - E-book management[8] and Calibre (software)[9]

Popular e-readers[10]

---

3. https://www.makeuseof.com/tag/android-ebook-reader-annotation/

4. https://computers.tutsplus.com/tutorials/
   beyond-highlighting-how-to-get-the-most-from-your-annotations--cms-20013

5. https://www.makeuseof.com/tag/annotations-guide-and-tools/

6. https://www.google.com/
   search?ei=kBpLXNi8M6jSjwTV_rDQDw&q=annotations+ebook&oq=annotations+ebook&
   gs_l=psy-ab.3..0i30j0i8i30l5.22647.24929..25651...0.0..0.114.1056.6j5......0....1..gws-wiz.......0i7
   1j0i7i30j0i67j0i10j0j0i8i7i30.F1Cm7BEmGFg

7. https://connect.ebsco.com/s/article/
   How-to-Print-E-mail-or-Save-EBSCO-eBooks-Pages-as-a-PDF?language=en_US

8. https://calibre-ebook.com/

9. https://en.wikipedia.org/wiki/Calibre_(software)

10. https://en.wikipedia.org/wiki/E-reader#Popular_e-readers

11. https://en.wikipedia.org/wiki/Comparison_of_e-readers

12. https://en.wikipedia.org/wiki/Comparison_of_Android_e-reader_software

13. https://en.wikipedia.org/wiki/Sigil_(application)

14. https://en.wikipedia.org/wiki/OverDrive_Media_Console

15. https://itstillworks.com/ereader-texttospeech-18619.html

Introduction

A few weeks ago, I had no idea I would be writing about Coronavirus (CV). Yes, it was going on in the world but I didn't pay much attention until it affected me personally. Wow, there have been such big changes in such a short time!

What got my personal attention was the new "Coronavirus Prevention Guidelines" for all of us. I understand the logic behind the guidelines, which are to protect us as we live our lives, especially as we "travel" from here to there. I see the new CV Guidelines as analogous to the travel procedures after 9/11[1] – inconvenient but necessary and do-able.

As our CV Precautionary Guidelines evolved, I thought something was missing. There was lots of talk about "Outside-In" strategies for Preventing and Treating CV, e.g. hand washing, social distancing, etc. On the other hand, I didn't hear and still don't hear much about the "Inside-Out" strategies for Preventing and Treating CV, e.g. boosting our Immune Systems.

Wearing Masks, Social Distancing, Hand Washing, etc. are "External Defenses" (outside us) against outside pathogens like the Coronavirus.

Inside us, we also have an "Internal Defense" System, which is commonly called our Immune System. Our Immune System is multi-dimensional, very complicated, inter-connected all throughout our body, and most incredibly works all by itself 24/7 with little or no outside interventions, most of the time. This book is geared toward doing what we can to keep the outside-outside – and to maximize our Immune System on the inside – thus creating a very powerful "Coronavirus Firewall".

---

1. https://en.wikipedia.org/wiki/September_11_attacks

I think we need both Outside-In and Inside-Out strategies for Preventing and Treating CV. By doing both Outside and Inside, we should have a better chance at fending off the Coronavirus and/or recovering from Coronavirus.

Let me say, that what you read in this book applies to just about any illness because every illness has an "Outside Component" and an "Inside Component".

IMPORTANT - Please follow your local guidelines for CV Prevention and Treatment. These guidelines are different around the world. Check with your local authorities.

The guidelines you usually hear about are the more common "Outside-In" strategies, e.g. hand washing and social distancing. This book is about the "Inside-Out" strategies that you might not hear elsewhere.

I will also cover briefly the usual "Outside-In" Medical Interventions, e.g. vaccines. In addition, I will cover a multi-dimensional Outside-Inside "Medical" Intervention that you might not have even considered.

I sure hope we have a Covid-19 Vaccine[2] someday. Development of such a Vaccine might take longer than what we figure and we will just have to learn to live with it, until then. What else can we do?

Please be sure to check out all the References for this book to give you background information.

****

OK, onward we go... (Isn't this exciting?)

---

2. https://en.wikipedia.org/wiki/COVID-19_vaccine

****

Take-Aways

- Boosting our Immune System is often overlooked in the Prevention and Treatment of many illnesses, including Coronavirus.
- By augmenting "Outside" Guidelines with Immune System Boosting, we have a better chance of minimizing the effects of Coronavirus on each of us.
- Why not do both Outside and Inside? What do we have to lose?

****

Got your attention? I hope so. Let's read more....

Chapter 1 – Coronavirus - The Inside Story

You've probably read lots about the Coronavirus[1] (CV) and current related Pandemic[2] related to Physical Health. This chapter covers what it is doing to our Mental Health.

Whether you have been diagnosed with Coronavirus or not, you have been infected by "Coronavirus On Your Mind". Think about it right now. Most of everything you want to do you can't do due to CV.

Here are some examples of how CV is affecting our everyday lives adversely and we can't do much about it at all, right now.

- We can't come near the people we want to be with;
- People are getting sick and sometimes dying all around us;
- Many of us can't go to work, have to adapt to working at home, or have no more job to go to;
- The world economy is deteriorating and our savings are diminishing;
- People are doing what they don't want to do, not trained for, not equipped with, etc.;
- We can't get what we want or need in the stores;
- Some of us have to make Decisions involving the Balance between Economy and Saving Lives. These decisions are not only business decisions, but they are also moral decisions;
- As a business owner, you might be worried sick how you will survive with fewer customers due to social distancing guidelines, less production due to worker distancing, possibly new OSHA rules, slowing down assembly lines, raw material

---

1. https://en.wikipedia.org/wiki/Coronavirus

2. https://en.wikipedia.org/wiki/2019%E2%80%9320_coronavirus_pandemic

shortages, more safety training, liability aspects, etc.;

- You might feel like you were "hit and run" and/or were robbed. What happened? It was so quick. What do I do now?
- Front line Healthcare Workers are putting their Emotions on Hold and more or less are having to "function as machines" to handle the influx of new patients;
- Primary Care Providers might be seeing an influx of patients with Chronic Conditions. Stress can cause/aggravate Chronic Conditions, e.g. Asthma, Irritable Bowel, Pain, etc. These comorbid conditions might be fertile ground for the Coronavirus to sprout, if the conditions/stress are not managed properly;
- Patients are being encouraged to use E-Visits, but this might be hard for some people – plus the Doctor just cannot do a "Hands-On" Examination over the phone and/or virtually;
- As Businesses and Schools start Opening Up - You're frustrated because you are following Guidelines and others are not (masks, social distancing, hand washing, etc.)
  - ○ You're a Healthcare Worker and are scared to death that you will be deluged with patients just like before;
  - ○ You're a Parent/Caregiver and you're scared that your loved one(s) will get sick due to the action/ inaction of others;
  - ○ You're a worker, now back at work, and you're scared that you'll be out of work again due to the action/ inaction of customers, co-workers, etc.
- You live with/care for a Person who is susceptible to CV and you both are scared to death;
- Whether you like it or not you are some Wave of this Pandemic, as illustrated in the "Health Footprint of

Pandemic" Graph in this article - Nursing and Post Pandemic Health Challenges[3]. Along with the Physical Aspects of CV, you might be experiencing the Fourth Wave in the graph....

- ○ Psychic Trauma;
- ○ Mental Illness;
- ○ Economic Injury;
- ○ Burnout;
- ○ In addition, a whole bunch more psychological/ emotional aspects of this pandemic we have yet to discover as a society.

- You might feel like you're walking on thin ice, checking the safety as you go, staying away from people who even look like they're sick, fearing you're exposing yourself to danger if you venture out in the world;
- You're an Essential Worker and yet you have a whole "bucket load" of feelings going to work;
- Yikes, public restrooms are closed! What's with that? Arggh:
- You're working from home and you just don't like it. It's too hard. You're afraid working from home might be the New Normal
- You're working from home and you do like it. It's great. You're afraid, sad, depressed thinking about going back to work the way it was;
- You might be falling more, making more mistakes, having accidents, "in a fog", etc. thinking and hearing about CV;
- Your Chronic Health Conditions might be more troublesome these days, worrying about CV, e.g. pain, stomach troubles, etc. Also, you seem to be catching more colds, infections are slow to heal, and/or feel tired most of the time;
- You're frustrated because you can't...

---

3. https://blogs.bmj.com/ebn/2020/04/15/nursing-and-post-pandemic-health-challenges/

- ○ Go where you want to go;
- ○ Do what you want to do;
- ○ Get what you want to get.
- You might be grieving over what was lost and what might be lost in the future. What happened to my nice life? Now it is gone and might not ever be the same again. You feel like "the rug has just been pulled out from underneath you" and there is no way out of this;
- You might be starting to think this is a hopeless situation, that there is no end in sight, and we'll have to live like this all the rest of our lives;
- You might just want to give up (please don't, though);
- You find yourself thinking of germs all the time now on anything and everything – and it's getting worse.
  - ○ If you become Hypervigilant[4], Obsessive-Compulsive[5], and/or Germophobic[6], please try to calm down and "get a grip". If unable to do so, please seek Professional Help. This is important.
  - ○ There is indeed a balance between CV Preventative Activities, e.g. hand washing, and Creating Undue Internal Stress. Let's face it. There are germs everywhere. There's only so much we can do without creating another problem, like Neurosis[7], or some other Mental Illness.
  - ○ Follow Local CV Prevention Guidelines, Relax, and Hope for the Best. By doing so, your Immune System will thank you.
- If you are an older person, have CV prone conditions, etc. –

---

4. https://en.wikipedia.org/wiki/Hypervigilance

5. https://en.wikipedia.org/wiki/Obsessive%E2%80%93compulsive_disorder

6. https://en.wikipedia.org/wiki/Mysophobia

7. https://en.wikipedia.org/wiki/Neurosis

are you "worried sick" you might get the Coronavirus?

- Do you live/care for someone who is susceptible to the Coronavirus? Are you on "pins and needles" worrying, protecting, cleaning, hovering, etc.?
- You might be micromanaging life, those you live with, your employees, etc. - for fear of something worse happening;
- You're at the breaking point and just can't handle anything else;
- "Essential Workers", e.g. Hospitals, Grocery Stores, Gas Stations, etc. might feel anxious and/or guilty about continuous exposure and the risk to themselves and their families;
- Even after we have a working CV Vaccine, what will life be then? It probably won't be the same. What will be the New Normal? How will I survive?;
- If you are working, you might be working harder and longer, due to lack of workers or due to increased load;
- You might be worried about whether your job will be there when you get back, if so how will my job change as a result of this;
- We have to wear these stupid face masks and wash our hands more;
- Our kids are at home, not in school, are bored, and it's really affecting me. Furthermore, I can't get to work to pay the bills;
- You may have had CV and/or Influenza and are scared stiff you will get sick again. You know you're Immune System is already weakened by your recent bout with CV, Influenza, or even the Common Cold;
- You're worried they might not ever get a CV Vaccine and we'll have to live like this forever;
- We can't do our favorite activities. We're bored. We used to have a good routine. We're stuck at home and every day is the

same, like the movie Groundhog Day[8];

- Maybe the greatest frustration of all is that other people aren't doing what they're supposed to be doing – following CV Guidelines. You're doing your part and others are not doing their part in this situation.
- In addition to CV, there are other troubling situations in the world, maybe even locally, that scares you and/or makes you sad. You might feel that you just can't take any more bad news!
- Most everyone is freaking out about something related to the current situations. Patience wears thin. It begins to look like there is no hope. Yuck!

Enough about that – What is above and much more is the problem. Now, what are we going to do about it?

Let's first look at what all the Stress is doing to our Immune Systems. It's well known that periods of intense and/or prolonged Negative Stress causes and/or aggravates Symptoms. If you don't believe me, look at the multitude of references on Stress in my previous book "Paging Dr. Within[9]" (Chapter 3). (This might look like a shameless plug for my other book, so be it. – I just don't want to repeat what I have already written!)

Anyhow, moving forward, let's now look at what blocks and/or fixes the Coronavirus in our bodies. It's our Immune System[10].

- Hand washing, social distancing, etc. all relate to blocking the CV from entering our bodies (external efforts);
- Our Immune System works to protect us Internally. A CV

---

8. https://en.wikipedia.org/wiki/Groundhog_Day_(film)

9. https://books2read.com/u/mBgJnA

10. https://en.wikipedia.org/wiki/Immune_system

Vaccine[11] (yet to be developed) trains our internal Immune System to detect and fight the CV pathogen.

So now, you see that our Immune System does the work on the "Inside Out", after all. We can help by following CV Precaution Guidelines and be Vaccinated when available. This is something we <u>can</u> do to help ourselves get better and stay better.

What more could we do? Let's work on both the "Outside In" and the "Inside Out". We've already talked about the Outside-In Stuff, so let's move on to what we can do from the Inside-Out. What we can do is Manage Stress and more importantly Manage the Stressors!

You've probably heard lots about Managing Stress[12], e.g. Meditation, Deep Breathing, Exercise, Prayer, Nature, etc. The above, and more, provides temporary respite. When we're done respiting, we're still back in the same situation, which we can't do much about. Nothing has changed, but we're calmer, which the Immune System likes. ☺

How do we stay calm long term? This amounts to Managing our Stressors[13], e.g. environment, chemical stressors, social stressors, and just plain Stress. Stressors are different for each person. Some things do not bother some people, whereas other people are stressed out to one degree or another.

You probably have lots of time now, so why not figure out what your Stressors are. Keep a log of your day, week, and maybe longer. See what bugs you; what worries you; what you cannot stand, etc. Your emotions will guide you in this. Years ago, we were often told not to show emotions. Well, that might be good in some situations, but long term it just creates more stress, like a pressure cooker ready to pop.

---

11. https://en.wikipedia.org/wiki/COVID-19_vaccine

12. https://en.wikipedia.org/wiki/Stress_management

13. https://en.wikipedia.org/wiki/Stressor

As you go along, note what makes you happy, sad, fearful, angry, etc.

From Vaudeville (Smith and Dale) [14] –

- SMITH: Doctor, it hurts when I do this.
- DALE: Don't do that.

So, what is this comedy routine telling us? Probably, don't do the things that hurt us, e.g. worry, hang onto anger, dwell in sadness, etc. Negative thoughts come and go, but we can choose how long we ruminate on those negative thoughts. With practice, it becomes easier to sweep negative thoughts away. Sometimes we might need extra help or education on how to do "mental housekeeping".

Before I forget, I should also mention that Negative Stress could cause and/or aggravate many illnesses. Think about it. Does worry, anger, etc. cause you to have more physical pain? This is because Stress is directly related to Pain. Another example is gastrointestinal distress. Because of this CV crisis, is your stomach touchier? All this relates to Mind-Body Stuff, which no one wants to talk about – both patient and doctor. Reminds you of the Elephant in the Room [15], doesn't it? Well, folks, there are many Mind-Body Interactions going on these days with this Pandemic. Did I say yet that Stress weakens the Immune System? No? Well, now I just said it.

Please note that this CV situation could very well develop into serious Mental Health Conditions [16] some of which are listed below. Please see professional help, better sooner than later. This book is not what you need at that time. This book is meant to offer up information on how to stay more or less in the "green zone" during this crisis. Mental health

14. https://en.wikipedia.org/wiki/Smith_and_Dale

15. https://en.wikipedia.org/wiki/Elephant_in_the_room

16. https://en.wikipedia.org/wiki/Mental_disorder

during the 2019–20 coronavirus pandemic[17] is a serious matter, which I'm wondering if we're prepared for.

The Physical Aspects of CV (sickness), if it occurs, has a beginning and an end – one way or the other. The Psychological/Emotional Aspects of CV vary by the day, week, month, etc. and might very well have long-term effects.

Many tragic events are short-lived, e.g. the September 11 attacks, Tornadoes, even Death of a Loved One. There is an end to it. This Coronavirus Situation has the potential of dragging on and on – for months, maybe more. This is Chronic Stress[18]. We might be Social Isolating, Hand-Washing, Distancing, Masking in Public, Staying at Home, etc. for a long time, sad to say. (Don't worry – I have good news later in this book.)

Mismanaged and/or Untreated, Chronic Stress can develop into more serious physical and/or mental conditions.

Furthermore, each person reacts/responds differently to the Coronavirus Situation.

- Social Isolation might not affect Introverts as much as Extroverts. Maybe "herding" or the desire to be near others might be part of our DNA or Survival Instinct. I don't know. I only know that now with Social Isolation, especially the lack of closeness, I feel lonely. What others and I do about this is in Chapter 3.
- People with greater Psychological resilience[19] might fare better than those more Sensitive and/or Rigid. This is related

17. https://en.wikipedia.org/wiki/
   Mental_health_during_the_2019%E2%80%9320_coronavirus_pandemic

18. https://en.wikipedia.org/wiki/Chronic_stress

19. https://en.wikipedia.org/wiki/Psychological_resilience

to "Resistance to Change".

Long term Coronavirus, or any other disaster, could lead to:

- Panic Attacks and/or Anxiety Disorders;
- Situational and/or Clinical Depression;
- Trauma and Stressor related Disorders, including PTSD;
- Somatic Disorders;
- Addictions, e.g. Alcohol, Drugs, Gambling, Food, etc.
- Sleep-Wake Problems;
- Family Problems, e.g. Children picking up Parent's Stress
- And, the list goes on....

Please, if you think you're having trouble coping, seek Professional Help.

Let's try to stay out of the Mental Health Danger Zone, if possible. That's what this book is about, in addition to keeping our Immune System happy and healthy to manage any CV pathogen situation.

Take-Aways

- Following CV Guidelines <u>and</u> improving our Immune System provides maximum protection against the physical and mental aspects of coronavirus.
- The decision is up to you. Follow CV Guidelines or not. Keep your Immune System healthy or not. The choice is up to you. You are responsible for your own health. An even small measure of "taking care of yourself" is beneficial.
- If you are a parent, you are also responsible for the health and well-being of your children. Do your best. In taking care of your children, don't forget about taking care of yourself, too.

Jump to this Chapters References or otherwise keep reading to go to the next chapter.

Chapter 2 – Let's Keep Our Immune System Happy and Healthy

Here's a Big Secret that you might not even hear from your Doctor.

Secret - *"Whether or not you get Coronavirus or not – and whether you recover/survive from Coronavirus – depends on Your Immune System."*

When we do get a Working Covid Vaccine, it only does so much. Vaccines[1] just "stimulates the body's immune system to recognize the agent as a threat, destroy it, and to further recognize and destroy any of the microorganisms associated with that agent that it may encounter in the future." Our Immune Systems do the "dirty work". Doesn't it make sense to have a Strong Immune System to begin with and use vaccines, as recommended?

- So, the first line of defense is to Maximize your Immune System to fight off anything and everything, e.g. Coronavirus, Common Colds, Influenza, Infections, etc.
- At the same time, Minimize Harmful situations from breaching your Immune System Barrier(s), e.g. mouth, nose, skin, etc. Please at least follow your local Coronavirus Prevention Guidelines. These Guidelines will keep you safe from other illnesses too, in addition to CV, e.g. Colds, Flu, etc.

Currently, we don't have an "Immune System Checker/Tester". Yes, we do have Lab Tests to show a more serious condition of Immunodeficiency[2], but nothing so far to show the condition of a

---

1. https://en.wikipedia.org/wiki/Vaccine

2. https://en.wikipedia.org/wiki/Immunodeficiency

Normal Immune System – Strong, Weakening, Weak. We can only go by certain Signs. Some signs of a Weak Immune System are below.

- You get sick more often, e.g. Frequent Colds;
- You have frequent Stomach/Bowel Problems;
- Your wounds are slow healing;
- You have frequent infections, e.g. ear/nose and often needing antibiotics;
- You are often tired, exhausted, and just feel worn out;
- You might need lots of medicines/treatments/doctor's visits;
- You have trouble sleeping;
- You're suffering from disease, illness, and maybe just with life.

Check with your doctor if you think you might have a Weak or Weakening Immune System. Your Doctor can look at the Bigger Picture in Diagnosis/Treatment. Ask what can be done to Maximize your Immune System.

This chapter describes the "care and feeding" of our Immune System, which we need more than ever right now.

Below are some objectives for Maximizing our Immune System.

- Good Sleep;
- Good Nutrition (Eat Right);
- Clean Air and Water;
- Good Sanitation;
- Moderate Exercise;
- Drink enough fluids, especially water;
- Use both "Stress Management" for short term relief and "Stressor Management" for longer-term relief and/or Prevention of Stress;
- Stay Positive and Hope for Better Days Ahead;

- Stay active. Keep your mind and body busy, but not too busy;
- Release your feelings/emotions when you can;
- Safe, Healthy, and Positive Social Interaction (within Coronavirus Social Distancing Guidelines)

Now, let's look at each of these as it relates to the Coronavirus Situation.

Tip – If our Immune System is in good shape, it can keep us safe from many maladies, in addition to CV.

****

Sleep

Scenario – You're in bed. It's time to sleep. The kids will get up soon – and you just can't sleep, worrying about things that the CV crisis caused. You already had enough things to worry about, now this! AAGH!

So, what can we do about it? (The next chapter further breaks down everything into possible Action Steps.)

- Try to relax. Easy to say, hard to do.
- Avoid eating too much before bedtime.
- Don't have stimulants before bed, e.g. caffeine, nicotine.
- Exercise during the day, but not too close to bedtime.
- Disconnect from technology a little bit before bed, e.g. turn off stressful TV programs, phones, computers, etc. – and do some relaxing, maybe even boring, things.
- Try to go to bed at the same time and get up about the same time each day, weekends included.
- Avoid naps after mid-afternoon.
- Avoid alcohol just before bed.

- Make your bedroom quiet, dark, cool, and comfortable – a place conducive to sleep.
- If all else fails, check with your doctor, if possible. Maybe they can help.

Good Nutrition

- Remember when your parent told you "Wash your hands before eating"? Well, they were right. We don't need any more germs for the Immune System to fight right now, do we?
- Eat as good, clean, nutritious food as you can, but not too much, or too little. You might have to check with a Healthcare Professional to learn how to eat, especially now to boost our Immune System. Many of us just don't know how and when to eat properly. We were never taught or shown how to do this. Maybe we were shown or taught and ignored it, for the most part. Well, now's the time to eat right for our own sake.

Clean Air and Water

- Avoid polluted Air and Water, e.g. Allergens, Smoke or Vape, Unsafe Water Supplies, etc.
- Get some fresh air, if possible.
- Maybe have your air and water tested to make sure it is safe. No need to burden your Immune System with something we can do something about.

Good Sanitation

- Please follow local CV guidelines for hand-washing and general cleanliness.

- Keep your environment clean. This applies to toilets/latrines, general housekeeping, etc.

Moderate Exercise

- If possible, try to get some outside exercise in the clean fresh air. It does a body good.
- Another word for Exercise is Physical Activity. This could amount to anything, depending on personal limitations, if any.
- Regular exercise is helpful for the body and mind in general. You even get to enjoy it.

Drink more Water

- Urine, Feces, and Breathing are the body's ways to get rid of toxins and other waste products. We might as well provide our bodies with what it needs to keep us in good health, all around.
- Our Immune System identifies pathogens, toxins, etc. and tries to get rid of them. By drinking more than adequate water, we ensure our "plumbing system" has what it needs to do its job.

Use both "Stress Management" for short-term relief and "Stressor Management" for longer-term relief and/or Prevention of Stress.

- This is a tricky one since you might have Past Stress/Trauma + Current Stress/Trauma + Future Anticipated Stress/ Trauma/Worry = Lots of Overall Stress - (which weakens the Immune System).
- Stress can originate...
    - Externally, e.g. Environmental, other people,

situations;

- ○ Internally, e.g. Worrying;
- ○ A Combination of Both External and Internal, e.g. Reacting Adversely to an Event, Situation, and/or a Person.

- Emotions and Intuition can help guide us out of Harmfully Stressful Situations.
    - ○ Listen to your Body.
    - ○ What does your gut tell you?
    - ○ How am I feeling around this Situation and/or Person?

- Stress Management – Relax – slow down, chill out, calm yourself down, loosen up, recline, sit back, unwind, chillax, take it easy, cool down, cool your jets, decompress, kick back, lighten up, mellow out, simmer down, take time to smell the roses, etc. However you relax is good, as long as it is done in a healthy manner.

- Stressor Management –
    - ○ Identify your personal Stressors – what bugs you; makes you mad; irritates you; what causes you pain/ discomfort; what irritates/aggravates/frustrates you; what inconveniences you; what do you think of as a nuisance; what troubles you; what do you often worry about; etc.?
    - ○ Minimize and/or Stay Away from your Stressors.
    - ○ Remember the earlier Vaudeville skit? – "Don't do that". Find a way to do something different instead of reacting to your Stressors. It's best to respond/act on Stressors, instead of letting them control you. Can you afford intense cumulative negative stress now at the risk of your own health?
    - ○ Then go relax after you've Managed Stressors. You

deserve a rest.

Stay Positive and Hope for Better Days Ahead, Whatever <u>Your</u> "Better" Might Be

- Important - Limit severely the amount of news you're exposed to via the Internet, TV, Family/Friends/Contacts, etc.;
- Look for the good in any situation at any time of the day. Look for the "Silver Lining[3]";
- Remember back briefly to when you got through tough times before;
- Humor heals and makes your Immune System happy. Did you ever hear of Norman Cousins[4] who used humor to heal himself? There's lots more out there on Positive Thinking - if you just switch from looking at "what's wrong" to "what's right", e.g. this oldie but goody – The Power of Positive Thinking[5];
- Did you know there is a whole field of study called Psychoneuroimmunology[6] that looks at how thoughts and emotions affect the Immune System? A Positive Attitude elicits a Strong Immune System. Having Hope is having a Positive Outlook for the Future.

Release your feelings/emotions when you can.

- Here are some good ways to release Negative Feelings or Emotions:

---

3. https://en.wikipedia.org/wiki/Silver_lining_(idiom)

4. https://en.wikipedia.org/wiki/
   Norman_Cousins#Illness_c0cb5f0fcf239ab3d9c1fcd31fff1efc__laugh_therapy_and_recovery

5. https://en.wikipedia.org/wiki/The_Power_of_Positive_Thinking

6. https://en.wikipedia.org/wiki/Psychoneuroimmunology

- Take a few deep breaths when you're stressed out. This provides temporary relief by triggering the Relaxation Response. This is particularly helpful when you are with others and don't feel safe being emotional.

- Do some writing about what is troubling you, what you are grieving over, how helpless you might feel, how frustrated you are, etc. Don't censor your writing as you go. Just write what comes into your head and feel the emotions as they come up. Cry, get angry, etc. I bet you'll feel better after doing this – physically and emotionally. Get it out, as much as you can. Your Immune System works better when you're not clogged up with a bunch of Negative Feelings (Stress).

- Exercise can help release pent-up emotions too. Let the emotions come out as you work out, run, walk, row a boat, punch a heavy bag, etc. It's good for your body and your mind to do so.

- Talk with someone, preferably who will just listen to you and not try to interrupt or "fix you". When you feel safe, talk about what is really going on – not chit chat about the weather, recipes, or sports – but rather get to a gut-level conversation. This talking might be with a good trusted friend and/or a healthcare professional, e.g. trained therapist.

- Sleep also can release emotions that you block during the day. Let them be. You can't control your dreams anyhow, so just sleep. Maybe it will look better in the morning or after a mid-day nap.

- Another emotion management opportunity might be watching movies, doing a creative activity, and/or listening to music. This can go both ways – it can help you release emotions and also help you get in a better mood.

- On the flip side, please don't do much or any of these:
  - Please don't deny that you think and feel as you do. You are you and your thoughts and feelings are valid for you. Do the same for others. Let others think and feel as they do;
  - Please don't withdraw, go inside yourself, isolate unnecessarily, or hide from life;
  - Please don't take it out on others, e.g. bullying, treating others badly, etc. – especially don't take it out on children and/or others who are vulnerable;
  - Please don't hurt yourself and/or others because of how badly you feel;
  - Please don't comfort yourself in unhealthy ways, e.g. excessive alcohol, drugs, food, gambling, work, etc.

Do Safe, Healthy, and Positive Social Interaction (within Coronavirus Social Distancing Guidelines)

- Probably the most important interaction, and often overlooked, is the "interaction with yourself".
  - Ask yourself - How are you feeling? What is my body telling me? What can I do about this? What are my options?
  - Then, be open for answers – "It's hard but you can do it", "Here are some options" "Go for a walk" "You're in good hands" "You've gotten through tough times before, like this"
- Beyond "talking with yourself" ☺ - Look for safe healthy social interaction opportunities –
  - Call someone and ask how they're doing. After

> hearing them, you might realize you're better off
> than you think;
> ○ Try something new – video conferencing, send a
>   pick-me-up card to a friend or family member,
>   learn/use new technology, etc.;
> ○ Innovate – try online gaming, take a virtual trip
>   with someone, use your "imagination" with another,
>   etc.

- I'd like to emphasize POSITIVE in whatever safe and healthy interaction you choose. The interaction should make you feel better, not worse. Don't hang around people or situations that make you feel bad. You can't afford negative interactions now since this is "stressful" and your Immune System doesn't like Stress.

Take-Aways

- Our Immune System likes it when you "Take Care of Yourself".
- Taking Care of Yourself is Multi-Dimensional.
- Maximizing your Immune System and Following CV Guidelines will give you the maximum "Viral Protection" available. In addition to fighting off CV, this combination will prevent many other illnesses, make you get better faster if you are sick, and stay better.

Jump to this Chapters References or otherwise keep reading to go to the next chapter.

Chapter 3 – So, What Can We Do About It ?

In the last chapter, we covered how to Maximize our Immune Systems from the "Inside-Out" to fight off Coronavirus and other dangers. Reviewing, here are the key points:

- Good Sleep
- Good Nutrition
- Clean Air and Water
- Good Sanitation
- Moderate Exercise
- Drink enough fluids, especially water
- Use both "Stress Management" for short-term relief and "Stressor Management" for longer-term relief and/or Prevention of Stress.
- Stay Positive and Hope for Better Days Ahead
- Stay active. Keep your mind and body busy, but not too busy.
- Release your feelings/emotions when you can.
- Safe, Healthy, and Positive Social Interaction (within Coronavirus Social Distancing Guidelines)

In addition, Please follow your local guidelines for CV Prevention and Treatment. These guidelines are different around the world. Check with your local authorities. These are "Outside-In" guidelines to thwart off pathogens before our Immune Systems see them.

Also, Please get a "Flu Shot[1]", sooner than later to better your overall chances of staying healthy and not unduly overload your

---

1. https://en.wikipedia.org/wiki/Influenza_vaccine

Immune System. Check with your Doctor on when to get a Flu Shot, as well as any other Vaccinations[2] needed for optimal health.

As I said earlier in this book, I think it's important to do both "Outside-In" and "Inside-Out" ways to help our Immune System. Some reasons to think so are:

- After we "Return to Normal/Work/School", we'll then be exposed to the Coronavirus more readily again. We might as well be prepared with our Inside-Out Immune System Maximization in addition to continuing to follow Coronavirus Guidelines (Outside-In).
  - This might be analogous to having our car checked/repaired before going on a long trip. We want to treat ourselves as good as our cars, don't we?
- Even after a COVID-19 vaccine[3] (Outside-In) is available, it probably will not be universally effective against all types of Coronavirus.
  - We run into that with Seasonal Flu Shots. These flu shots are better than nothing, but they only reduce the risk of getting the flu by 40-60%, according to the CDC.
  - It just makes sense, at least for me, that any vaccine will have a better chance of working if the person's Immune System is in good shape to begin with (Inside-Out).
- Coronaviruses are here to stay, in their various forms, probably until we develop a Universal Coronavirus Vaccine. Even then, Viruses are sneaky little fellas who are prone to mutating into another variation, not covered by the CV vaccine of the day.

---

2. https://en.wikipedia.org/wiki/Vaccination_schedule

3. https://en.wikipedia.org/wiki/COVID-19_vaccine

○ So why not gird up our Immune System (Inside-Out) to defend us against CV bugs, as well as other diseases. We might as well have 360-degree protection, just like our Computer Virus Software, which protects against a multitude of computer viruses and other malware.

○ Did you know that Coronaviruses are one of the causes of the Common Cold[4]? Hmmm?

****

One huge thing we can do is ask our Doctors for a "Personalized Coronavirus Prevention & Action Plan" – just tailored for you! Some things you and your Doctor might discuss are below.

- *Based on my overall health, what are my chances of getting CV* if I follow the Current Local General CV Prevention Guidelines? – e.g. from CDC, WHO, State Governors, etc.
   ○ Should I do more Preventative Measures beyond the General Guidelines, based on my current health conditions? – e.g. Asthma or other Breathing Diseases, Heart Disease, Diabetes, etc.
   ○ What should I do regarding my Mental Health, during this crisis, based on my history? – e.g. Susceptibility to Depression, Anxiety, etc.
- *Based on my overall health, what are my chances of recovering and/or dying from CV, if I do get it?*
   ○ What can I do to improve my chance of recovering?
- *What CV Symptoms should I watch for, considering my current health conditions?*
- *If I do see CV Symptoms, what should I do, considering my current health conditions?*

---

4. https://en.wikipedia.org/wiki/Common_cold

- *Should I be tested for Coronavirus? If so, how do I do that?*
- *What should I do when the Coronavirus Restrictions lift?*
  - *What should I do when I go back to work? Can I do the same job I did with Coronavirus around? Do I need a Doctor's Slip based on my health? What Protective Equipment should I wear at work? – Is this practical for the work I was doing? What other CV guidelines should I follow at work?*
  - *What should I do when I go back to school? Do I need a Doctor's Slip based on my health? What Protective Equipment should I wear in school? – Is this practical for my school and studies? What other CV guidelines should I follow in school?*
- *What can I do about all the Coronavirus Stress I'm having? How can I help myself?*
- *What can I do personally to Improve my Immune System?*
- *Is there anything else I should be concerned about at this time? – or can I just follow your Personalized Advice, Relax, Do what I can, and Hope for the Best?*

If you are a Care Giver/Taker, you can also ask your Doctor(s) for a "Personalized Coronavirus Prevention & Action Plan" for both you and whom you care for. Don't forget about you, when caring for others! Remember on airlines, they say to put on your oxygen mask first then assist others? This applies here too. If you go down, then you won't be able to help anyone.

Each member of the family/household should get a "Personalized Coronavirus Prevention & Action Plan" for at home and when they go back to work/school/public areas, etc. – e.g. Parents should get "Personalized Coronavirus Prevention & Action Plan" for each their children, especially for when the children go back to school.

Given a "Personalized Coronavirus Prevention & Action Plan" by your Doctor, now decide what you're going to do about it.

You can choose to do what is best for you and your children/ dependents, despite what others do or don't do around you.

- Set Realistic Goals for you and your children/dependents/ family going forward. Use Common Sense.
- Modify as you go. Re-evaluate as you go.
- Don't give up.
- Live life as much as you can, staying safe and healthy.

****

Another thing we can do about this is to monitor our Stress Levels. We do have a built-in way of doing this, by monitoring our emotions. Chapter 2 covered how too much negative stress, especially cumulative, can affect our Immune Systems, amongst other body functions.

The problem is that many of us ignore and/or suppress our emotions for one reason or another. This is not good long-term. Yes, we probably have to put our emotions on hold short-term sometimes, but it is good to acknowledge and/or release our emotions long-term. If not, these unhandled or mishandled emotions might lead to physical and/or mental symptoms. Some common illustrations are below.

- I just can't stomach this situation.
- That person is a pain in the neck.
- I have a tension headache.
- You make me sick.

Before these types of symptoms, we receive an early warning that "something is not right". Ignoring or suppressing our Emotions is much like ignoring or taping over the Check Engine Light in our car.

So, what goes on beyond the symptoms? Internally, our Immune System is working overtime and being burned out because we're not taking care of ourselves. Our Immune Systems weaken with too much long-term negative stress. It can handle short-term stress quite well, but long-term is not so good.

What happens when our Immune System is weak? We get sick.

Now, what can we do about monitoring our Emotions to keep our Immune System Healthy and Happy?

- We can learn to monitor our own emotions from the inside out. You know when you're angry. You know when you're carrying a Grudge. You know when you're fearful, anxious, etc. You also know when you're stressed out.
- We can also monitor our emotions from the outside, too, via technology. An example of this is this article - Getting all emotional: Wearables that are trying to monitor how we feel - It's not just Amazon that's exploring emotion-sensing wearables.[5] I predict that Monitoring Emotional Stress and/or Pain will be routine in the future for both Patients and Healthcare Workers, e.g. Doctors, Nurses, etc.
- Your Immune System will thank you if you use Stress Management to relax short-term and Stressor Management to handle/avoid harmful situations/people long-term. Chapter 1 discussed Stress/Stressor Management. You can also refer to the References at the end of this book.

****

---

5. https://www.wareable.com/wearable-tech/wearables-that-track-emotion-7278

I'm bored and lonesome. How about you? What can we do, beyond all this Outside-In and Inside-Out talk? (Reminds me of an Innie or Outie Belly Button) ☺

During this time, below are some ideas of what to do to keep busy, stay healthy, and be as happy as we can be. I hope you find these helpful. Please remember to follow local Coronavirus Guidelines in doing some of these, however.

- <u>Write a book</u>, like me – on anything! (Did I tell you I was bored? I don't want to bore you, but I really am bored. Are you tired of listening to me?) ☺
- <u>Connect</u> with Friends and/or Family. Make new acquaintances in your field of interest. Use Skype, FaceTime, Zoom, Google Hangouts, Marco Polo, etc. video chatting. Also, just calling on the phone means a lot to you and the person you are calling.
- **<u>Aagh – I Can't Stand This!</u>** – If you are having major troubles coping, please contact a Healthcare Professional. This book is not what you need right now. Might these be helpful for you?
  - Mental Health and Coping During COVID-19 | CDC[6]
  - Mental Health - Home Page - CDC[7]
  - Mental Health[8] – World Health Organization
  - Mental health and COVID-19[9] – World Health Organization

---

6. https://www.cdc.gov/coronavirus/2019-ncov/daily-life-coping/managing-stress-anxiety.html

7. https://www.cdc.gov/mentalhealth/index.htm

8. https://www.who.int/mental_health/en/

9. http://www.euro.who.int/en/health-topics/health-emergencies/coronavirus-covid-19/novel-coronavirus-2019-ncov-technical-guidance/coronavirus-disease-covid-19-outbreak-technical-guidance-europe/mental-health-and-covid-19

- <u>Stop, Look, and Listen</u> – As long as you are stopped, due to no cause of your own, would it be a good time to re-evaluate your life?
  - Think about it...are you doing what you want to do in life?
  - Ask your family, how you are doing. Maybe your family likes you being home more and would be willing to forego some luxuries to have you home more.
  - Were you hiding in your work due to a bad home life?
  - Is/Was your Work getting you down and adversely affecting your Health?

Talk to yourself first, and then talk with those who you live with. Talk it over. Strive to help each other be what all of you want to be in life.

See which direction you all want to go in after social isolation.

Do you want to go back to what you did? On the other hand, do you want to make a change?

Who says you can't? If it's okay with you and those you live with, care about, etc. – Why not?

Plan what you all want to do with the rest of your life. On your mark, get set....then just wait for GO!

- <u>Read</u>. Library buildings are closed but online services are still available, e.g. e-books, e-zines, etc.
- <u>Calm Down</u> – Meditate, try Guided Imagery, even Self-

Hypnosis. You can do this by yourself, with others via video-conferencing, and/or online videos.

- Thank "Essential Workers" – by words and/or actions – e.g. Healthcare Workers, Police/Fire, Grocery Stores, Gas Stations, etc.
- Check with your doctor on when to get a Flu Shot, as well as any other vaccinations for yourself and your children. Your Immune System might be overloaded battling both Influenza and Coronavirus. No sense unnecessarily overloading our Immune Systems when we can do something about it.
- Make Yourself and Essential Person by attending to essential services in your life, e.g. doctor's appointments, self-care, continuing physical/mental therapy, getting prescriptions, etc. If you have trouble taking care of your essential needs, ask for help, and/or look for solutions in another place. Do what you can using technology, e.g. virtual visits, but sometimes you and someone else just have to be in the same place at the same time. One example of this is an in-person visit to a doctor to do a hands-on examination you just can't do over the phone or in an e-visit. Common sense prevails. Take care of yourself and you'll be in a better spot to help others, if need be.
- Get and/or Buy "Peace of Mind". For example - Connect with a Budget Counselor[10]; Ask your Doctor to explain CV and how it relates personally to you and your family. Taking care of your "Inside" might very well help your "Outside" feel better, i.e. symptoms. For me, I'm spending more on Cell Phone Minutes because I feel better talking to others – it brings me peace of mind – and sometimes after hearing them talk too, I realize I don't have it so bad after all.
- Brainstorm ideas with others on how to solve/overcome the

---

10. https://en.wikipedia.org/wiki/Credit_counseling

CV problems. You can do this casually at a distance and/or use Computer supported Brainstorming Tools[11].

- <u>Start</u> preparing yourself and your children for going back to work and/or school.

Have plans based on the current CV Prevention Guidelines and/or your Doctor's Personalized Guidelines mentioned earlier in this chapter.

- How are you and your children going to follow the Guidelines at work/school? – e.g. Face Masks, Social Distancing, Hand Washing, etc.
- How will you and your children deal with possible teasing and/or bullying by others, e.g. other workers/students, bosses, schools, employers, etc.?
- You and your children can prepare yourself now and be ready when you can go back to work/school. It's better to prepare than to "wing it" with safety/health.
- Figure out a way for you and your children to stay safe/ healthy at work/school balancing what "should" be done with common sense.
- Empower yourself and your children to "take care of yourself" despite what others are doing or not doing. Encourage yourself and your children to do what's best for you. Your health/safety is up to you and your children – your actions/inactions are a decision you can make.

- <u>Make</u> your own Home Altar[12], Meditation Space, a place to "get away from it all" and maybe get a better perspective of what's going on and what to do about it. If sick, maybe it would help to make a Healing Machine[13], Healing Prayer

---

11. https://en.wikipedia.org/wiki/Computer_supported_brainstorming

12. https://en.wikipedia.org/wiki/Home_altar

Focalizer[14], Healing Cookies[15], etc.

- <u>Look</u> outside your own little circle where you live. See people around the world going on with their lives despite poverty, sickness, wars, etc. See children playing, people going to work, people hanging out the wash, folks playing chess in the park, people gathering around, etc. – *all doing as best as they can, despite the troubling situations around them.* Learn from them. Do what you can to keep on living. Don't let this situation get you down.

- <u>Take</u> Care of Yourself and those you live with. Do what you all need to do to stay healthy, safe, sane, and maybe even happy – for yourself and those who need/depend on you. Prevent Getting Sick[16]. If you're sick in some way, do all you can to get better and stay better. If you're sick with CV, follow local Guidelines and/or check with your Doctor. What to watch for - Symptoms of Coronavirus[17] Click on this link If You Are Sick or Caring for Someone[18].

- <u>Find</u> Someone to Listen to you – just listen, not fix, just listen. Do the same for others. Answers will come once you get the problem out in the open. Children and Elders need someone to just listen, too. This Someone might even be a Pet, a squirrel in the park, someone/something beyond you, a chatbot, whatever works- and you will feel better afterward. Writing helps get things out too. Don't hold in your feelings

13. http://interesting-health-information.blogspot.com/2014/08/how-to-make-your-own-healing-machine.html

14. https://thevirtualhealingmachine.blogspot.com/2015/12/healing-prayer-focalizer_18.html

15. http://interesting-health-information.blogspot.com/2014/09/15-ideas-on-how-to-make-healing-cookies_15.html

16. https://www.cdc.gov/coronavirus/2019-ncov/prevent-getting-sick/index.html

17. https://www.cdc.gov/coronavirus/2019-ncov/symptoms-testing/symptoms.html

18. https://www.cdc.gov/coronavirus/2019-ncov/if-you-are-sick/index.html

– get them out appropriately in some way or another.

- <u>Plan</u> what you're going to do in the "New Normal" of the day, week, month, maybe for the rest of your life. Pick and choose who and what you want in <u>Your</u> New Normal". Is this CV Lockdown a "Wake-Up Call"? Question what you did/didn't do before CV and see whether you want to continue them. Rebuild your life today for <u>your</u> tomorrow. Start anew. Consider this situation as a New Start, a Reboot, or something like that. Ask yourself –

    ◦ Do I want to go back to spending what I did before CV lockdown?

    ◦ Do I want to go back to the same job?

    ◦ What do I want in my "New Life"? Whom do I want in my "New Life"?

    ◦ Do I want to go back to what I was doing before all this started? Do I <u>really</u> want to? Do I have to? What are my options?

    ◦ Do I want to rebalance my Work-Life/Family Routines going back? What is really important to me going forward? Was I in a "rut" before, just going to work day after day going nowhere? What do I want to do now and in the future?

    ◦ What do I need/want to do to take care of myself and my children in the New Normal?

- <u>Start and/or Join</u> Coronavirus Groups on Social Media, e.g. Facebook – for whatever you want or need – support, information, solutions, etc. Please try to stay away from anything Negative at this time. Your Immune System is bogged down already with all the Negative News. Give your Immune System a break by "feeding it" positivity, good solutions, feeling not alone, etc.

- <u>Look</u> at the Big Picture around any Symptoms you might be having – physical and/or mental symptoms. Your symptoms might be caused/aggravated by all the Stress you're under. Talk this over with your Doctor to see how much of your symptoms are related to stress vs. something else, either physically and/or mentally. Might these Stress Resources be helpful for you? If you manage your Stress or better yet your Stressors, maybe your symptoms will improve or even go away.

- ○ Mental Health and Coping During COVID-19 | CDC[19]
- ○ Mental Health - Home Page - CDC[20]
- ○ Mental Health[21] – World Health Organization
- ○ Mental health and COVID-19[22] – World Health Organization

- <u>Make</u> a way for children/elders to report abuse during this time.
  - ○ With schools being out, children are home, thus not observed by teachers who usually report child abuse;
  - ○ Similarly, children in schools have ready access to counselors to "talk things out" – again not readily available with school being out;
  - ○ With social isolation, elders might be mistreated and no one around to help them report it.

- <u>Grieve</u> your losses in this Pandemic. All of us have lost something in this event and it might be ongoing. You might be grieving the loss of a loved one, the loss of your job, the

---

19. https://www.cdc.gov/coronavirus/2019-ncov/daily-life-coping/managing-stress-anxiety.html

20. https://www.cdc.gov/mentalhealth/index.htm

21. https://www.who.int/mental_health/en/

22. http://www.euro.who.int/en/health-topics/health-emergencies/coronavirus-covid-19/novel-coronavirus-2019-ncov-technical-guidance/coronavirus-disease-covid-19-outbreak-technical-guidance-europe/mental-health-and-covid-19

loss of time spent with loved ones, the loss of financial security, etc. Grief is usually not a one-and-done deal – it takes time – and sometimes comes and goes. Don't let grief get you down, though. Maybe some of these links will help you grieve.

- Grief and Loss[23]
- Loss and grief amidst COVID-19: A path to adaptation and resilience[24]
- Funeral Guidance for Individuals and Families[25]
- Death of a Colleague During the COVID-19 Pandemic Understanding and Managing Grief for Healthcare Workers and Leaders[26]
- Complicated Grief: What to Expect After the Coronavirus Pandemic[27]
- Managing Bereavement around the Coronavirus (COVID-19)[28]
- Relearning ways to grieve[29]
- Trauma, moral injury, and grief[30]
- The little losses caused by COVID-19 add up. Here's how to deal with them.[31]
- Why feelings of grief and loss are normal during

23. https://www.cdc.gov/coronavirus/2019-ncov/daily-life-coping/stress-coping/grief-loss.html

24. https://www.ncbi.nlm.nih.gov/pmc/articles/PMC7177068/

25. https://www.cdc.gov/coronavirus/2019-ncov/daily-life-coping/funeral-guidance.html

26. https://files.asprtracie.hhs.gov/documents/death-of-a-colleague-during-covid.pdf

27. https://www.ncbi.nlm.nih.gov/pmc/articles/PMC7264152/

28. https://complicatedgrief.columbia.edu/wp-content/uploads/2020/04/Managing-Bereavement-Around-COVID-19-HSPH.pdf

29. https://news.harvard.edu/gazette/story/2020/04/learning-how-to-mourn-during-a-pandemic/

30. https://psychiatry.ucsf.edu/coronavirus/coping#f

31. https://www.startribune.com/the-little-losses-caused-by-covid-19-add-up-here-s-how-to-deal-with-them/569723612/

COVID-19[32]
- ○ Grieving life and loss[33]
- ○ Understanding Grief in the Age of the COVID-19 Pandemic[34]
- ○ Coronavirus Has Upended Our World. It's OK To Grieve[35]
- ○ SAMHSA – Coronavirus (COVID-19)[36]
- ○ Grief[37] and Kübler-Ross model[38] and Anticipatory grief[39]
- ○ Libraries usually have self-help books on how to work through grief. Check with your local librarian.
- ○ If you're having trouble with grief and/or any other mental/emotional health issue, please seek help.

- Check out Support Groups[40]. Soon, I'm sure there will be CV Support Groups to help those who are struggling in one way or another from Coronavirus. It's important to "tell it like it is", to talk about feelings, and to not feel alone during a crisis.
- Help yourself and maybe others with CV Self-Help[41] Resources. There are more and more Self-Help Books[42] and

32. https://wexnermedical.osu.edu/blog/why-feelings-of-grief-and-loss-are-normal-during-covid19

33. https://www.apa.org/monitor/2020/06/covid-grieving-life

34. https://www.verywellmind.com/understanding-grief-in-the-age-of-the-covid-19-pandemic-4801931

35. https://www.npr.org/sections/health-shots/2020/03/26/820304899/coronavirus-has-upended-our-world-its-ok-to-grieve

36. https://www.samhsa.gov/coronavirus

37. https://en.wikipedia.org/wiki/Grief

38. https://en.wikipedia.org/wiki/K%C3%BCbler-Ross_model

39. https://en.wikipedia.org/wiki/Anticipatory_grief

40. https://en.wikipedia.org/wiki/Category:Support_groups

41. https://en.wikipedia.org/wiki/Self-help

other resources geared to Coronavirus, like this book you're reading now. Check on Google Books[43], Book Sellers/Stores, Worldcat[44], etc.

- <u>Make</u> a list of what's bothering you today with the CV and ongoing in life. Prioritize what bothers you the most, then start working on that list to resolve things, rather than just worrying and ruminating over things. Taking action, however small, will make you feel better. Your Immune System likes it when you feel good.

- <u>Take</u> care of the big stuff first, e.g. make a new budget, look for a new/temporary job, be nice to your children, etc. Work on what bothers you the most. Keep pecking away at it. If you can't do the big stuff now, do some smaller stuff first to get warmed up, and then tie into the tougher items.

- <u>"De-Lonely"</u> yourself and others. Reach out to people you forgot about. Ask them how they are doing. You and the other person will both feel better. Maybe Connect2Affect[45] will help you get started and/or give you more ideas.

- <u>Focus</u> on **You** and **Your Children**, not on what others are doing or not doing. You have control over yourself and your children. Others are going to do what they're going to do or not do. You take care of yourself and your children to stay safe, healthy, and happy.

- <u>Stand</u> up for yourself and your children. Be and Set a good example for your children, now and for later in their lives, on how to take care of themselves, no matter what.

- <u>Teach/Show/Encourage</u> your children to express their Emotions in Healthy and Appropriate Ways. Show and Lead

---

42. https://en.wikipedia.org/wiki/Self-help_book

43. https://books.google.com/

44. https://www.worldcat.org/

45. https://connect2affect.org/

by Example. Your Children have to "let it out" as much as you do. Stifling, downplaying, suppressing Emotions is just not healthy. Teasing and Bullying those who are emotional is harmful. Everyone of any age has Emotions around this CV Situation – old, young, or anywhere in between. No one has the answers. We're all doing the best we can. Once you or your children "get it out in the open", you'll probably feel better, and can start finding solutions to what is bothering you and/or your children.

- <u>Read</u> CV Self-Help Books to help yourself and your loved ones. New ones are being published daily. These books might give you some good information, tips, hope, etc. to get through this. There's something for everyone. Your local library might be able to suggest books for you, too.
  - For Parents[46];
  - For Children[47];
  - How to Cope[48], in general.

---

46. https://www.google.com/
search?tbm=bks&ei=I5q9XqLILIO4tQaPqKHQDA&q=%28coronavirus+OR+covid+OR+pandemic%29+parents&oq=%28coronavirus+OR+covid+OR+pandemic%29+parents&gs_l=psy-ab.3...19100.24637.0.25321.31.20.0.0.0.0.256.2663.0j12j5.17.0....0...1c.1.64.psy-ab..18.3.567...33i10k1j33i299k1.0.33CYiWPDXGo

47. https://www.google.com/
search?tbm=bks&ei=Ppq9XujPD5iStAaZ74P4CA&q=%28coronavirus+OR+covid+OR+pandemic%29+%28children+OR+kids%29&oq=%28coronavirus+OR+covid+OR+pandemic%29+%28children+OR+kids%29&gs_l=psy-ab.3...98057.106167.0.106891.25.25.0.0.0.0.140.2448.8j15.23.0....0...1c.1.64.psy-ab..2.5.606...33i299k1.0.e53UTmROY4A

48. https://www.google.com/
search?tbm=bks&ei=F5u9XpX7C8m6tAbiho3gCA&q=%28coronavirus+OR+covid+OR+pandemic%29+%28struggling+OR+cope+OR+coping%29&oq=%28coronavirus+OR+covid+OR+pandemic%29+%28struggling+OR+cope+OR+coping%29&gs_l=psy-

- <u>Say</u> "play uplifting music" to your Alexa, Google Home, Siri, etc.

- <u>Hire Yourself Out</u> as a Remote Worker (Work-from-Home) - to help kids with their schoolwork, just listen to you or your children, to be an Administrative Assistant to others working from home, etc. – whatever you think you can do. Check on the Internet to see how others are Working Remotely. Also, check Freelance Sites like Fiverr[49] and Upwork[50], which has workers all around the World working remotely.

- <u>Take</u> two pieces of paper. On piece #1, list what you **can do** during this CV time. On piece #2, list what you **cannot do** during this CV time. Throw piece #2 away. Keep piece #1 and get going on some things you **can do** during this CV time.

- <u>Appreciate</u> what you have today. Appreciate your freedom, albeit somewhat limited. Appreciate that you're alive and plan to stay that way. Appreciate those around you. Appreciate you do have a life, even with these limitations now.

- <u>Give Up</u> the fantasy that things will go back to <u>exactly</u> the way they were before CV, anytime soon. Instead, hold on to what you do have today and see what "tomorrow" brings. Imagine "tomorrow" is an unopened gift – what's inside? Wait and see. In any event, you can handle it and maybe even enjoy the New Tomorrow someday.

- <u>Make</u> it a better day today, instead of hoping for better days in the future. We really don't know what the future will bring. What can you do to make it a better day today? Then, act on it. Make it a good day. Protect your good day from negative

---

ab.3...9611.32053.0.32868.49.40.0.0.0.0.155.4205.12j27.39.0....0...1c.1.64.psy-

ab..14.12.1433...33i299k1j33i10k1.0.T5Pnj-UP5-0

49. https://www.fiverr.com/

50. https://www.upwork.com/

people, news, situations, etc.

- <u>Watch</u> what you say to others. Before you open your mouth, you have a choice of whether you spread positivity, hope, encouragement – or spread unnecessary fear, worry, gloom, doom, etc. In these times, might it be good to err on the positive side? By the way, if you're thinking all those negative thoughts, your Immune System doesn't like that. Our Immune System thrives on positive things, excitement, hope, dreams, etc.

- <u>Don't</u> let CV "eat you alive", especially from the Inside-Out by Unhealthy Coping Mechanisms, e.g. Depression, Addictive Behaviors, Worry, Stress, etc. Act and/or Respond to CV Difficulties instead of Hiding from or Reacting to CV Problems. Your Immune System likes Positive Actions/ Responses and dislikes Negative Reactions to any situation.

- <u>Talk</u> with your children about CV, using age-appropriate wording of course. Maybe they know more than you think.

  - Let them express their emotions, if any. They must see your worry, everyone wearing masks, etc.;

  - Re-assure them that you are doing everything you can to keep them safe;

  - Don't expose them to undue negativity, but rather talk hope;

  - Let them know what is expected of them regarding following CV Prevention Guidelines;

  - Remind them to let you know if they're not feeling well – that it's best to catch things early – and their symptoms are probably not CV, but rather a common cold or something like that;

  - You might also monitor your children, as well as yourself, for stress-related symptoms, e.g. upset stomach, fatigue, insomnia, depression, etc.

All the above might apply to those you live with, care for, etc. that have dementia or some other kind of mental disorder/limitation, too.

In essence, keep an open-dialogue going to know about "what else is going on" with those you live with and/or care for. People might not have CV Physical Symptoms (Outside) but might very well have lots going on the "Inside".

- <u>Change</u> your attitude, your perspective, and/or your expectations. If you're having trouble doing so yourself, consider seeing a Therapist, Counselor, Life Coach, etc.
- <u>Focus</u> on what you can do, not on what you can't do. It is what it is, right now – get over it, get on with life as best as you can now, get going and do what you can.
- <u>Work</u> on what bothers you the most, e.g. financial situation, getting groceries safely, getting healthcare for your children, etc. Do what you can short-term and let the long-term happen when it happens – then you can deal with that. No need to worry about the long-term now, since you don't know the future – no one really does. If you can't fix/change "it" right now, leave "it" alone, and fix/change what you can. You probably have enough to do, just fixing/changing things you can. Ask for help as needed or wanted. Keep going. Keep moving forward. Don't let it get you down. Your Immune System likes positive action(s) and dislikes worry, frustration, etc. You need to have your Immune System strong now. Some resources to help you resolve what's bothering you the most are below. Take Charge of your life as it is and you will feel better.
  - Call 211[51] in the U.S. and Canada – "...to provide

51. https://en.wikipedia.org/wiki/2-1-1

information and referrals to health, human, and social service organizations...";

○ Crisis Hotline[52];

○ National Suicide Prevention Lifeline[53] - "...National Suicide Prevention Lifeline (1-800-273-TALK [8255]) is a United States-based suicide prevention network of 161 crisis centers that provides a 24/7, toll-free hotline available to anyone in suicidal crisis or emotional distress...";

○ Help with Bills | USAGov[54]

○ Call 911[55] in North America – "...for use in emergency circumstances only..." Also, see List of emergency numbers[56] (worldwide);

○ Hesperian Health Guides[57];

○ Also, check the References at the end of this Chapter. You don't have to be miserable or feel helpless in any situation. Ask for help. It's okay and you'll feel better afterward knowing that you took action on your problems. Others can give you hope when maybe you see no hope at all. What do you have to lose by asking for help or just asking someone to listen? We're all in this together. No one is exempt from CV stress. Everyone is affected adversely in some way or another. You're not alone. ☺

• Pet the Pet. Walk the dog. Play with the Kitty. You would be

52. https://en.wikipedia.org/wiki/Crisis_hotline

53. https://en.wikipedia.org/wiki/National_Suicide_Prevention_Lifeline

54. https://www.usa.gov/help-with-bills

55. https://en.wikipedia.org/wiki/9-1-1

56. https://en.wikipedia.org/wiki/List_of_emergency_telephone_numbers

57. https://hesperian.org/

surprised how relaxing being with animals is. Your pets will like this too. ☺

- <u>Just Say No</u> to unsafe and/or unhealthy situations and/or people. If you are an Essential Worker[58], think about what you're doing and whether you want to continue as-is or make changes. The same goes for a bad home situation for yourself and your children. Think of yourself and your family. Your family needs you to be healthy, alive, and present as much as you can. Don't act rashly, if you don't have to. Think about it. Think about the bigger picture - not just your work, your career, and/or money. Talk about it with others, especially your family. Maybe consider counseling to help you make decisions on what to do or not do. You alone can decide what is best for you and your family (children). Maybe there's something better for you. ☺

- <u>Plan</u> now how you will fit into the "New Normal" after CV. Yes, there will be a new normal. Things just won't be the same. When you think about it, life is a series of "New Normals". So what can you do about it? Learn about what might change in your life after CV – and plan how you might adapt. There are references at the end of this book on CV New Normals, but at this time, it is only speculation. Whatever comes, you can fit yourself into it – or not. Maybe you don't have to participate in some aspects of the New Normal. You are in charge of your own life and the lives of your Children.

- <u>Choose</u> to "take good care of yourself", following Preventative Guidelines, much like you <u>Choose</u> to take care of your car. You <u>choose</u> to have regular oil changes and other maintenance in your car - why not give yourself that same consideration? In many locations, CV Prevention Guidelines

---

58. https://en.wikipedia.org/wiki/Essential_services

are not mandatory. Thus, in most areas each person <u>chooses</u> to follow – or not follow – the local Guidelines. It's up to you to <u>choose</u> what is best for you and your family. For me, I'm <u>choosing</u> Health by following Guidelines. The <u>choice</u> is up to you too.

- <u>Judge Not</u> others for what they do or don't do. You have the <u>Right</u> to <u>follow</u> CV Preventative Guides, just as others have the Right to <u>not</u> follow Guidelines, in most localities. You're not the "Covid Police". Getting upset about other's actions/ inactions does nothing good for you or the other person – it just makes your Immune System upset and you don't need that now. Until it becomes a habit, you might have to gently remind yourself to "Mind Your Own Business". ☺

- <u>Think</u> about good memories instead of worrying. Think of all the money you're saving staying home. Think of how you can help others from a distance. Think about how you're "building character" in your children by dragging them out of the house to go for a walk. Think of what's good about CV and maybe share this with others.

- <u>Consider</u> the upsides of the CV Guidelines – probably less chance of getting Colds, Flu, etc. Think of how you can turn the CV Guidelines into Opportunities, especially if you are out of work – make customized face masks, offer yourself as CV Guideline Trainer for when Businesses/Schools open up, make medical devices to remind people to follow CV Guidelines, etc.

- <u>Post</u> good positive thoughts/messages on social media. Find good news about CV and share it on social media. Do your part to counteract all the negative in the world right now. You never know how your little action might perk someone up or even "make their day". Send smiley faces to your contacts. Post and/or share Positivity on Social Media via

posts, comments, pictures, etc. Here are a few starters...
- ○ Positive Energy+[59]
- ○ Power of Positivity[60]

- <u>Draw</u> an uplifting picture or message at the end of your driveway. Humor helps too.

- <u>Make</u> peace with someone or something. "Mend fences" in relationships, if you can, if it doesn't hurt you or the other person. Forgive someone or yourself. Your Immune System will thank you for doing any or all of these. It was expending energy with all this negative thinking and acting. Your Immune System wants to run efficiently and not waste energy or healing power on unnecessary internal stress.

- <u>Do</u> random acts of kindness. Leave a flower or positive note on someone's porch. Let them know they are appreciated just for being alive.

- <u>Old People Unite</u> – Let's show these young 'uns how healthy we can be – physically, mentally, and emotionally.

- <u>Make</u> a Newsletter, News Page, Publication of Good News, what's good about CV, interviews with positive people, etc. You might not make any money doing this but you might make someone feel better – and in doing so, you feel better too.

- <u>Look</u> outside your little life sphere. See how the birds are making nests? Nature doesn't listen to the news. Nature gets on with life. Let's do the same. Yes, nature sometimes has to adapt to the current situation, e.g. climate change, storms, etc. They just do it. Let's do the same. Move on. Keep living. Do what you need to do today – and make it a good day.

- <u>Stop</u> thinking, worrying, ruminating, and go do something (within CV Guidelines). Take action on something you want

---

59. https://www.facebook.com/positiveenergyplus/

60. https://www.facebook.com/powerofpositivity/

to do or something that has been bothering you.

- <u>Keep</u> busy, positive, moving ahead, hoping. It makes you feel better when you have a sense of control over something. An example of this is Patient Controlled Pain Relief[61].
- <u>Play</u> Bingo, Games, etc. – at home with those you live with and/or virtually using the Internet.
- <u>Hope</u> for a better tomorrow. Do what you can to make it a good day today. Spread hope with others. Smile at others. Cheer others on. Did you know that Hope is contagious? Despair is contagious too. Let's choose Hope today.
- <u>Act</u> Young, if you are an older person. Think like a Young Person. Go on with your life, as best as you can. Stop thinking about your age, aches, pains, etc. Take some healthy risks. Your Immune System likes to "feel young", too.
- <u>Attend a Religious Ceremony</u> via video-conferencing and/or online videos.
- <u>Do</u> a Virtual Workout, Dance Practice, etc.
- <u>Smile</u> and maybe chat with someone when you're out and about, maintaining social distancing, of course. You'd be surprised how good this alone feels.
- <u>Paint</u> rocks or pebbles, leave them in various places on your travels, and imagine someone finding them, maybe years from now.
- <u>Coffee Klatch</u> with others via video-conferencing, on the phone, etc. Depending on current local CV Guidelines, this might be possible in a park, again maintaining social distance.
- <u>Maintain Social Distance</u> around You and Your Children when out in a public setting. Either move yourself and/or ask the other person to move. Speak up if you need to. This goes for at work, at the gym, in church, in stores, etc. Also, goes for your children at school, at play, etc. Show your children how

---

61. https://en.wikipedia.org/wiki/Patient-controlled_analgesia

to do this. Be a good example. Be tactful and yet achieve this distancing. If distancing is just not possible, then it is doubly important to wear a mask. Do what you can and need to do to keep yourself and your children safe, healthy, and happy. Don't let others tease and/or bully you into not taking care. Your Immune System needs you to take care of it and protect it from unnecessary toxic situations.

- Ask others to cover their cough, if they don't do so. This might be hard for you since some may take offense. It's important though to be "out of the line of fire", even if it is your boss, co-workers, family, etc. From your actions, your children might learn how to take care of themselves, too.

- Go fly a Kite! – even if no one tells you to do so. ☺ Make your own kite, maybe using some of the links below.
  - Take Flight With a DIY Kite[62]
  - How to Build and Fly a Box Kite[63]
  - Easy Paper Kite for Kids[64]
  - How To Make A Kite - 27 Kites! Step-By-Step Instructions[65]

- Find Something via Dowsing[66], Metal Detecting[67], your Psychic Abilities[68], etc.

- Mail something to someone. Send a funny card to perk up someone's day, a care package to someone, a thank-you card, a "thinking of you" note, etc.

- Shop, Shop, Shop – Watch this one, if you're on a limited

62. https://www.pbs.org/parents/crafts-and-experiments/take-flight-with-a-diy-kite

63. https://boyslife.org/hobbies-projects/projects/53339/build-and-fly-a-box-kite/

64. https://www.instructables.com/id/Easy-Paper-Kite-for-Kids/

65. https://www.my-best-kite.com/how-to-make-a-kite.html

66. https://en.wikipedia.org/wiki/Dowsing

67. https://en.wikipedia.org/wiki/Metal_detector

68. https://en.wikipedia.org/wiki/List_of_psychic_abilities

budget now, though. Still, you can find lots of enjoyment from online shopping. Look for free things, if that's what you like to do. Get/Buy "junk", re-purpose it into art or something else, and maybe sell it on the Internet.

- <u>Have</u> Fun at whatever you like to do. Try something different and see if you like it.
- <u>Declutter</u> – Clean house, find good homes for unused items, downsize, etc.
- <u>Revive an Old Skill and/or Interest</u> – Maybe you were good at a musical instrument, Morse code, juggling, etc.
- <u>Learn a New Skill and/or Interest</u> – There are many online courses, some of which are available through your local library, e.g. Gale Courses[69]. You can get personal distance teaching by Freelancers and/or Online Teachers. You can find these instructors on the Internet. Fiverr[70] is one of many Freelance Services for just about anything. Furthermore, there is a plethora of free Learning Information on the Internet, as shown in this list of open online course providers[71].
- <u>Do something creative</u> – Cook, Bake, Draw, Sketch, Sculpt, Dance, Woodworking, Metal Art, etc.
- <u>Grow Something</u> – Start a garden. Weed a garden. Grow something on your windowsill. Plant a tree.
- <u>Home Schooling</u> – This might be necessary for parents now with children out of school. Have you ever thought of teaching others what you know via the Internet? How about helping others do what they want to do via video-conferencing?
- <u>E-Visit</u> a Museum. Here are 12 World-Class Museums You

69. https://www.gale.com/c/gale-courses

70. https://www.fiverr.com/

71. https://en.wikipedia.org/wiki/List_of_MOOC_providers

Can Visit Online[72]

- Explore your old neighborhood via Google Maps and Google Earth. Drive around virtually without even leaving home! Find new fishing/hunting spots. Find archeological digs.
- Work from home – For necessity and/or for fun, fulfillment, and/or just to keep busy. Search online for opportunities, as well as Freelance Websites, e.g. Fiverr.[73]
- Rearrange, Build, Tear Down, Modernize, etc. your living space. Make a hide-away, she-shed, man-cave, office, etc. all in your own backyard, apartment, patio, home.
- Exercise – by yourself and/or with others via video-conferencing, videos, etc.
- Look for the Good - Treasure Hunt. Purposely sleuth out what you're grateful for, your blessings, your talents, what you *do* have, etc. Go on an actual Treasure Hunt.
- Bury something without marking where it is and try to find it a week or so later (just for fun), etc. Bury a real Time Capsule[74] with your children and/or grandchildren, just for fun. Create a Pandemic Time Capsule With Your Kids[75], FREE Quarantine Time Capsule Printable for Kids[76], How to make a time capsule to remember this unprecedented time[77], etc.
- Bury/Burn your resentments and be done with them.
- Watch television, a movie, a bird making a nest, the sun rise and set, the waves coming in, the people go by, etc.
- Listen to the radio, to each other, to the sounds of silence, to

---

72. https://www.mentalfloss.com/article/75809/12-world-class-museums-you-can-visit-online

73. https://www.fiverr.com/

74. https://en.wikipedia.org/wiki/Time_capsule

75. https://offspring.lifehacker.com/create-a-pandemic-time-capsule-with-your-kids-1843109937

76. https://whatmomslove.com/kids/quarantine-time-capsule-printable/

77. https://www.cnn.com/2020/04/09/cnn-underscored/covid-19-time-capsule-ideas/index.html

crickets chirping, etc.

- <u>Eat Special</u> – with candlelights, on a picnic, in a boat in a mote - wearing a coat – inviting a goat – and that's all she wrote. ☺
- <u>Attend</u> an online concert, performance, etc.
- <u>Volunteer</u> using your skills at home, on the phone, via the Internet, etc. It doesn't have to be formal. Find little ways to help others. In doing so, you might forget about yourself and your troubles. Maybe your troubles will melt away, at least for a while, when you see how you helped someone else – see them smile and/or see them doing something they couldn't do before you came along, etc.
- <u>Groom</u> yourself and maybe those you live with. Give each other haircuts, manicures, massages, etc.
- <u>Play</u> games at home and/or online.
- <u>Make</u> a new Routine, since your old routine is gone for now. Adapt to the <u>current</u> New Normal. This short-term New Normal might be around for a while, and then it will change into a longer-term New Normal. Make the most of the day and be happy and healthy. Be productive.
- <u>Open</u> the Drapes and maybe the Window. Let the light and fresh air come in. Take some deep breaths of fresh air. Stick your head out the window a little bit. Listen to the birds. Don't be any more of a hermit than you have to be. Look at the world outside your little room, apartment, house, etc. See what you can do, then do it.
- <u>Do</u> puzzles, crosswords, etc.
- <u>Talk/Act</u> Positive - Fake it if you have to. Maybe you'll feel better by acting positive, upbeat, healthy, and happy.
- <u>Make</u> a CV Proof Moat around your house. Mark on your face mask "Coronavirus Stay Away". Instead of a Welcome Mat outside your house, get one that says "Stay Away".

I'm just kidding. ☺ The point is to try to lighten up a serious situation. Humor does help and the Immune System likes a light-hearted mood.

You could, however, make a book of Coronavirus Absurd Ways of Managing. I'm sure there's lots of weird coronavirus related things you could put in such a book.

- Put together a Jigsaw Puzzle, a Model Boat/Plane/Car, etc.
- Solve this List of unsolved problems in mathematics[78]
- Help create a coronavirus vaccine - This puzzle game lets you help create a coronavirus vaccine[79]
- Make wine, cheese, beer, maple syrup, cookies, candles, a breadcrumb trail for someone to follow you, etc.
- Organize your photos, music albums, fishing tackle box, etc.
- Sew, Knit, Fabric Art, Quilt something for yourself and/or others. Some people are making Face masks for both professional and personal use.
- Learn a new language, a new skill, how to play the piano, how to better maneuver through your life, etc.
- Camp out in your own backyard, living room, basement, etc.
- Find leaves, animal footprints, rocks, fossils, the meaning of life (Answer – 42), etc.
- Buy and/or Make a memento album, rock collection, coin collection holder, etc.
- Search for aliens, bigfoot, etc. or at least do some stargazing.
- Go geocaching, go out on a limb, get lost, go down a different street, go up to someone and smile/say hi, etc.
- Draw a masterpiece at the end of the driveway, an uplifting message on the sidewalk, draw air in and out (this is called

---

78. https://en.wikipedia.org/wiki/List_of_unsolved_problems_in_mathematics

79. https://thenextweb.com/corona/2020/03/05/puzzle-game-lets-you-help-create-coronavirus-vaccine/

breathing), etc.

- <u>Fix</u> your bicycle, your car, your faulty phone, etc.
- <u>Hangout</u> with people you like, that make you feel good about yourself, that have similar interests, are challenging for you in a good way – via phone, online, social media, video-conferencing, etc. Conversely – minimize contact with those who cause you negative stress. You can't afford optional negative stress right now.
- <u>Fly</u> a Plane, SpaceShip, etc. via Online Flight Simulators. The best free flight simulators[80]
- <u>Paint</u> by number, do finger painting, paint your house, paint those rusty chairs, do body painting, etc.
- <u>Create</u> a website, a blog/vlog, and/or a YouTube video/channel, etc.
- <u>Make Money</u> off CV? Yes, there are people making money off this situation. Do you want to? Do you need to, maybe to make ends meet?
  - ○ I hear of people sorting through old clothes, belongings, and selling them or giving them away. Depending on your location, you might be able to do curbside pickup from buyers.
  - ○ Search for Coronavirus on all of the Craigslists using SearchTempest[81] – to see what others are doing. This might give you some ideas. Also, check Amazon and eBay too.
  - ○ Search Freelance Sites for Coronavirus. Some examples are Fiverr[82] and Upwork[83]. Also, check out Etsy[84] if you're handy making things.

---

80. https://www.digitaltrends.com/gaming/best-free-flight-simulators/

81. https://www.searchtempest.com/

82. https://www.fiverr.com/

83. https://www.upwork.com/

- ° Stock Market Buys/Sells? – if you know what you're doing.
- ° Check out Google Patents[85] and PATENTSCOPE[86] for Coronavirus. Lots of ideas, devices, methods, and apparatus.
- ° Can you write, draw, make, invent, sculpt, create, etc. about Coronavirus?
- ° What services might you do related to Coronavirus?
- ° Some places are hiring in this CV situation. Look locally for "Hiring Signs". Check Job Services where you live. Check on LinkedIn. Also, check online job search engines. Temporary Employment Agencies might also be worth a try.
- ° Network...ask around....surf the net...see what others are doing to make a profit or at least make a living.
- ° What <u>can</u> you do while still observing your local CV Prevention Guidelines?

- <u>Get dressed up</u> and take selfies, or have a romantic dinner for whom you live with, etc.
- <u>Make</u> a fairy garden, an herb garden, grow tomatoes on your windowsill, grow a tree from a seed, etc.
- <u>Make</u> a collage from scraps of paper/cloth, photos, etc.
- <u>Color</u> a coloring book, color your hair, change the color of your bedroom, etc.
- <u>Start</u> a conversation with someone new on Tumblr or Twitter.
- <u>Repurpose</u> unwanted items to new items for your own enjoyment, as gifts, or sell them online.
- <u>Look</u> for a new job, a different job, a part-time job, a

---

84. https://www.etsy.com/

85. https://patents.google.com/

86. https://www.wipo.int/patentscope/en/

temporary job, a volunteer opportunity, a work-at-home job, a consulting gig, a freelance opportunity, etc.

- <u>Make</u> jewelry from anything handy around the house.
- <u>Be</u> gentle with yourself and others around you. This is a big thing. Don't expect too much out of yourself or others right now. We had no warning of this – we didn't get a CV Owner's Manual – and we all don't know what we're doing. We're all at a great loss of what to do and how to take care of ourselves and others. We're kind of at the mercy of others and the virus right now. *Pandemics just don't happen very often!*
- <u>Make</u> a fort out of pillows, blankets, tarps, ladders, furniture, etc.
- <u>Bring</u> the outdoors indoors. Make an indoor-outdoor garden. Open the windows and let some fresh air in. Pull up the shades.
- <u>Beautify</u> your house/apartment, yourself, your living partners, your pets, your car, etc.
- <u>Listen</u> to podcasts of your interest.
- <u>Try</u> making podcasts of your own. What do you have to lose?
- <u>Surf</u> the web for topics of your interest. Jot down what you find. Make a mind-map[87] of your finds to find more of the same. Use a thesaurus to find synonyms for your search terms.
- <u>Use</u> binoculars or a telescope for distance watching of people, birds, insects, etc. Conversely, use a magnifying glass or microscope to explore the hidden world right around you.
- <u>Tinker</u> around, fix something, or make something.
- <u>Putter</u> around the yard or house. Clean the Putter in your Golf Bag.
- <u>See</u> what can be home delivered – groceries, medications, merchandise, food, services, etc.
- <u>Daydream</u> about a vacation, a future event, the pleasant past,

---

87. https://en.wikipedia.org/wiki/Mind_map

etc.

- <u>Do</u> micro volunteering[88].
- <u>Record</u> audiobooks for those who need them. Read for LubriVox[89]
- <u>Hug</u> yourself and those you live with. Tell them how much they're appreciated.
- <u>Practice</u> yoga, the flute, standing on your head or doing cartwheels, etc.
- <u>Read</u> books, comic books, e-books, etc. Try reading books humorous to you. Humor heals and builds up the Immune System.
- <u>Be</u> around positive, upbeat people. Look for them. Avoid negative people and situations, now more than ever.
- <u>Have</u> an Italian day, a German day, an African day – eat the foods of the region, listen to their music, imagine that you're there, try to speak the language, etc.
- <u>Sing</u> as you've never sung before. Sing just for you. Let others think what they want. Be respectful, however to your living partners. Find a place where you can just be you and sing. Sing with others if they want to.
- <u>Make</u> musical instruments out of what you can find at home. You could be a one-person band or others could join you in a jam session with their own homemade musical instruments.
- <u>Install</u> a better TV antenna and/or expanded TV streaming device[90]. Check out free/paid program streaming services[91].
- <u>Get</u> an eBook reader. Check out eBooks through your local library, buy them online, and/or get Free eBooks[92]

---

88. https://en.wikipedia.org/wiki/Micro-volunteering

89. https://librivox.org/

90. https://en.wikipedia.org/wiki/Digital_media_player

91. https://en.wikipedia.org/wiki/Streaming_service_provider

92. https://wiki.mobileread.com/wiki/Free_eBooks

- <u>Upgrade</u> your router for faster gaming, streaming, video-conferencing, etc.
- <u>Project</u> your TV, smartphone, computer onto a wall and make a home theater. Is the popcorn ready, yet?
- <u>Do</u> karaoke with those you live with. Play charades. Perform a skit at home and share it via the Internet with family and/or friends. Make a YouTube Video of your liking.
- <u>Make</u> your own coffee blend. Roast your own coffee. Maybe make your own coffee enhancer.
- <u>Make</u> a meal from scratch. Make your own bread. Use ingredients around the house to make a unique meal. There's even Road Kill Cuisine[93]!
- <u>Plan</u> a wedding, your next trip, an ideal date, what you want to do with the rest of your life, etc.
- <u>Bake</u> Dandelion Cookies.
- <u>Make</u> meals to freeze for when you do go back to school and/or work. Be prepared, as some say.
- <u>Make or Buy a Chef's Hat</u> and make your own Sushi, French Pastries, etc. Act as if you know what you're doing. Pretend. Use your imagination if you have no talent. Practice on those you live with....or NOT ☺
- <u>Make</u> your own Health Club in the basement or a spare room. Use what you have around the house for weights and other exercise equipment – or order online to be delivered. You might not want to flood your basement for a swimming pool, however. You might hear about it! ☺
- <u>Invent</u> your own board game, patent it, and maybe sell it. Monopoly[94] got started that way.
- <u>Tune</u> out the world and meditate or just enjoy the silence. You could use earplugs, noise-canceling headphones, or just

---

93. https://en.wikipedia.org/wiki/Roadkill_cuisine

94. https://en.wikipedia.org/wiki/History_of_the_board_game_Monopoly

go to a quiet place. Maybe you'll get a better perspective of your life, find peace amongst all the angst going on, or even get a good nap.

- <u>Take</u> a bubble bath, take a break, take five, take a powder, take it all in, or take it as it comes.
- <u>View</u> online Tutorials to learn something or just for fun. Here is a Funny Example - Reddit's Vague But Funny Tutorials Teach You Nothing at All[95]. Seriously, though, you can learn so much online these days in whatever you're interested in.
- 100 useful things you can do to kill boredom if you're quarantined at home because of coronavirus[96]
- List: 100 things to do while stuck at home social distancing[97]
- 101 FUN Things to do in Isolation[98]
- 100 things to do when you're self isolating, social distancing & bored at home[99]
- 34 productive things to do at home during self-isolation[100]
- 50 things to make staying home easier while social distancing[101]
- 100+ Fun and Educational Things To Do at Home[102]

95. https://lifehacker.com/reddit-s-vague-but-funny-tutorials-teach-you-nothing-at-1796519722

96. https://i-d.vice.com/en_uk/article/n7jk77/100-things-to-do-quarantine-home-coronavirus-self-isolation-social-distancing

97. https://www.kvue.com/article/news/entertainment-news/things-to-do-in-self-quarantine/269-f002dfab-7edb-42cd-bc67-857b671dea1e

98. https://www.123homeschool4me.com/101-fun-things-to-do-in-covid-19-isolation/

99. https://www.youtube.com/watch?v=ztNwq27plow

100. https://www.racv.com.au/royalauto/living/at-home/things-to-do-home-self-isolation.html

101. https://www.usatoday.com/story/tech/reviewedcom/2020/03/17/50-things-you-need-stay-home-while-social-distancing-during-coronavirus-outbreak/5057159002/

102. https://www.plasticpollutioncoalition.org/blog/2020/3/27/100-fun-and-educational-things-to-do-at-home

- 50 Fun Things To Do When Bed Bound/House Bound[103]
- 10 Things You Can Do Today to Combat Senior Isolation[104]
- <u>Think Before You Act</u> on anything you see or hear. There are many Coronavirus Gimmicks, Books, as well as what others are doing or not doing these days. Think for yourself and your children. If something doesn't look or sound right, check it out. Don't just do or buy things because "everyone else is doing it". Regarding Health Claims, Products, Advice, etc. check with your Doctor to see if it is right for you. The same goes for this book, too.
- <u>Continue</u> following Local and/or Personalized CV Guidelines until your Doctor says it is safe to lessen or stop doing so. This is important even after you recover from CV, have been tested CV Positive with no Symptoms, and/or you receive a working CV Vaccine. Your Doctor is in the best position to advise you, because of the following:
  - ◦ After you recover from CV, your Immune System might be weakened to the point where you might get CV back again or get some other malady, maybe even worse than CV. It might be better to continue CV Prevention Guidelines until your Immune System is back up to its Normal Fighting Status for you;
  - ◦ If you have been tested CV Positive and yet have no Symptoms, your own Immune System might still be weakened. In addition, if you are CV Positive you probably are a Carrier of CV and can spread it to others if you don't follow CV Guidelines;
  - ◦ Yes, it is very important to get the working CV Vaccine, when and if it becomes available – *if it*

---

103. https://healing-boxes.com/50-fun-things-to-do-when-bed-boundhouse-bound/

104. https://www.aplaceformom.com/blog/6-20-16-things-you-can-do-to-combat-senior-isolation/

makes sense to you and your Doctor. Let your Doctor advise you whether the new CV Vaccine is right for you. Some Doctors like to wait a while to see how new Medical Interventions work out. You might not be a good candidate for the new CV Vaccine because of your other health conditions considering the possible CV Vaccine Side Effects. Your Doctor will look at the bigger picture around your overall health and decide whether the benefit of the new CV Vaccine is greater than the possible risks. Lastly, the CV Vaccine might not be 100% effective, similar to the efficacy of our annual Flu Shots. Trust your Doctor to act in <u>your</u> best interest.

- <u>Encourage/Motivate</u> others to follow CV Prevention Guidelines.

Some examples you might relate to are - your child just won't wear a mask – your customers won't wear masks and socially distance, yet you don't want to drive away customers – people with dementia can't or won't follow guidelines – Public Health Workers, Healthcare Workers, etc. are probably frustrated because people just aren't taking care of themselves in this Pandemic – etc.

Below might be some strategies to encourage/motivate people to follow CV Guidelines.

- Lead by example.
- Check around to see how others are managing a similar situation, e.g. other parents, schools/daycare centers, other stores/restaurants, your own doctor/therapist, government agencies, organizations, Behavioral Psychologists[105], etc.

---

105. https://en.wikipedia.org/wiki/Psychology#Behavioral

Below are some resources you might find helpful and there are a few more links in the References for this Chapter.

- What To Do When People Don't Practice Social Distancing[106]
- Army project explores ways to encourage protective COVID-19 behaviors[107]
- Coronavirus (COVID-19): Helping Kids With Autism Cope[108]
- 5 Tips to Help You Talk to Your Older Parents About Social Distancing[109]
- 7 Guidelines for Parents Sharing Custody of Children During the COVID-19 Pandemic[110]
- Considerations for Schools[111]
- Guidance for Child Care Programs that Remain Open[112]
- Keep Children Healthy during the COVID-19 Outbreak[113]
- Considerations for Memory Care Units in Long-term Care Facilities[114]
- Preventing the Spread of COVID-19 in Retirement

106. https://www.npr.org/sections/coronavirus-live-updates/2020/04/28/846684162/what-to-do-when-people-dont-practice-social-distancing

107. https://www.army.mil/article/235151/army_project_explores_ways_to_encourage_protective_covid_19_behaviors

108. https://kidshealth.org/en/parents/coronavirus-autism.html

109. https://www.healthline.com/health-news/talking-to-your-parents-about-the-importance-of-social-distancing

110. https://www.wardandsmith.com/articles/7-guidelines-for-parents-sharing-custody-of-children-during-the-covid-19-pandemic

111. https://www.cdc.gov/coronavirus/2019-ncov/community/schools-childcare/schools.html

112. https://www.cdc.gov/coronavirus/2019-ncov/community/schools-childcare/guidance-for-childcare.html

113. https://www.cdc.gov/coronavirus/2019-ncov/daily-life-coping/children.html

114. https://www.cdc.gov/coronavirus/2019-ncov/hcp/memory-care.html

Communities and Independent Living Facilities (Interim Guidance)[115]
- Standing Too Close. Not Covering Coughs. If Someone Is Violating Social Distancing Rules, What Do You Do?[116]
- Social distancing: How to persuade others it works[117]
- The Psychological Reason Why Some People Aren't Following COVID-19 Quarantine Orders[118]
- Effective health communication – a key factor in fighting the COVID-19 pandemic[119]
- Why so many people are still going out and congregating in groups despite coronavirus pandemic: It's not selfishness[120]
- Using psychology to encourage long-term COVID-19 compliance[121]
- Study Looks at Attitudes Toward Social Distancing in COVID-19 Pandemic[122]
- Increasing Adherence To Covid-19 Guidel Ines: Lessons From Existing Evidence[123]

115. https://www.cdc.gov/coronavirus/2019-ncov/community/retirement/guidance-retirement-response.html

116. https://time.com/5819816/coronavirus-social-distancing/

117. https://www.bbc.com/future/article/20200402-covid-19-how-to-convince-others-social-distancing-works

118. https://www.forbes.com/sites/briannawiest/2020/04/08/the-psychological-reason-why-some-people-arent-following-covid-19-quarantine-orders/#b9981e069054

119. https://www.ncbi.nlm.nih.gov/pmc/articles/PMC7180027/

120. https://thehill.com/changing-america/opinion/488654-why-so-many-people-are-still-going-out-and-congregating-in-groups

121. https://artsandsciences.osu.edu/news/psychology-long-term-covid-19-compliance

122. https://www.american.edu/spa/news/study-looks-at-attitudes-toward-social-distancing-in-covid-19-pandemic.cfm

123. https://www.povertyactionlab.org/sites/default/files/Lessons_health_evidence_increasing_adherence_COVID-19_guidelines.pdf

- Enforcing compliance with COVID-19 pandemic restrictions: Psychological aspects of a national security threat[124]
- Non-pharmaceutical public health measures for mitigating the risk and impact of epidemic and pandemic influenza[125]
- CDC Guidelines - Communities, Schools, Workplaces, and Events - Information for Where You Live, Work, Learn, and Play[126]
- There is much more on encouraging/motivating, generally and specifically for CV – check with your local librarian to help you find more. I hope you find something that works for you and your situation.

Underlying all this is the reluctance of some people to "take care of themselves" and/or "change their behavior" for their own health and for those around them. Some people are like that and probably won't change. You can try to encourage and that's about all you can do. For your own sake and sanity, you might have to make peace with how others are/aren't and get back to just taking care of yourself.

Please don't sit and fret. Fussing, fuming, etc. are harmful to the Immune System. Try to find a solution that works for you. Your Immune System will like that.

The main thing – Figure out a way to Cope/Thrive in a Healthy Positive Manner, not harm others by doing so, and not let it get you down.

---

124. https://reliefweb.int/report/world/enforcing-compliance-covid-19-pandemic-restrictions-psychological-aspects-national

125. https://apps.who.int/iris/bitstream/handle/10665/329439/WHO-WHE-IHM-GIP-2019.1-eng.pdf?ua=1

126. https://www.cdc.gov/coronavirus/2019-ncov/community/index.html

After reading this long list, I hope I brought at least a smile to your face and got you to be thinking of how to make the best of this situation. That's what I was aiming for. You might now think that life is not as bad as you thought – at least for today.

If you do get sick and are concerned, please call your doctor.

Take-Aways

- There is much you can do about it – whatever "it" is for you.
- Look for your options, search out your options, expand your vision, and don't stay stuck as a Victim of the Coronavirus Situation – or any other Situation. See what others are doing and how they are coping in a healthy positive manner. Learn from them.
- Your Immune System thrives on Healthiness and Positivity and is adversely affected by Negativity and Lack of Self-Care. Choose to be Positive/Healthy and your Immune System will thank you. ☺

Jump to this Chapters References or otherwise keep reading to go to the next chapter.

Chapter 4 – Coronavirus Treatment Information

Until we get a working Covid-19 Vaccine[1], we're all just dependent on the Condition of Our Immune System. After we do have a working Vaccine, it might not be available for all people for one reason or another, so we're still dependent on our Immune System.

Even with a Vaccine, whether it works or not for the individual is dependent on the overall shape of the Person's Immune System. Injecting a Vaccine into someone with a Weak Immune System will not guarantee Success. Our Immune System seems to do all the work in Recovery. Vaccines[2] only attempt to "teach" or "coax" our Immune Systems to recognize the Covid-19 Virus as a threat and "take care of it".

There are Coronavirus Treatments even now without a Vaccine, some of which are below. In addition to what is below, check the references for this Chapter. The word "accepted" below mostly refers to Treatment Recommendations from the CDC and/or the World Health Organization. I've also included experimental, alternative/complementary, unproven, etc. "Treatments" also in an effort to be complete (at the time of this writing).

"Accepted" and Alternative/Complementary CV Treatments:

- *Yes, by all means, get the Covid-19 Vaccine when it becomes available! – if it makes sense to you and your Doctor. Your Doctor can advise whether the vaccine is right for you.*
  - Keep in mind, however, that Vaccines are not always 100% effective. Vaccine Efficacy[3] depends on lots of

1. https://en.wikipedia.org/wiki/COVID-19_vaccine
2. https://en.wikipedia.org/wiki/Vaccine

factors. For example, Influenza Vaccine[4] is about 50% effective. COVID-19 drug development[5] researchers are doing their best, but the Coronavirus[6] is a "moving target" – Viruses have a nasty habit of mutating into "something else".

- At the time of this writing, much of CV Treatment is Experimental, as shown by the following:
  - COVID 19 Landscape of experimental treatments[7]
  - Information for Clinicians on Investigational Therapeutics for Patients with COVID-19[8]
  - COVID-19 Studies from the World Health Organization Database[9]
  - Exploring alternative medicine options for the prevention or treatment of coronavirus disease 2019 (COVID-19)- A systematic scoping review[10]
  - Research Into Traditional Remedies For COVID-19 Welcomed By World Health Organization[11]
  - Traditional Chinese Medicine in the Treatment of Patients Infected with 2019-New Coronavirus (SARS-CoV-2): A Review and Perspective[12]

---

3. https://en.wikipedia.org/wiki/Vaccine_efficacy

4. https://en.wikipedia.org/wiki/Influenza_vaccine

5. https://en.wikipedia.org/wiki/COVID-19_drug_development

6. https://en.wikipedia.org/wiki/Coronavirus

7. https://www.who.int/publications/i/item/covid-19-landscape-of-experimental-treatments

8. https://www.cdc.gov/coronavirus/2019-ncov/hcp/therapeutic-options.html

9. https://clinicaltrials.gov/ct2/who_table

10. https://www.medrxiv.org/content/10.1101/2020.05.14.20101352v1

11. https://healthpolicy-watch.org/research-into-traditional-remedies-for-covid-19-welcomed-by-world-health-organization/

12. https://www.ncbi.nlm.nih.gov/pmc/articles/PMC7098036/

- What makes things worse is that there is lots of Misinformation related to the COVID-19 pandemic[13] and Unproven methods against COVID-19[14]. **Generally don't do any of these unproven methods and don't believe any of this misinformation.** *If you have any questions, ask your doctor.*
- There are current CDC and WHO Treatment Guidelines, but these guidelines might change by the time you read this book.
  - Interim Clinical Guidance for Management of Patients with Confirmed Coronavirus Disease (COVID-19)[15] – CDC.
  - Coronavirus disease (COVID-19) technical guidance: Patient management[16] – WHO.
- It seems to me Healthcare Professionals are "doing what they can with what they've got" – to keep the CV Patient alive, as comfortable as possible – and hoping that the CV Patient's Immune System is able to fight it off.
- As a Reminder, please also get your annual "Flu Shot[17]" better sooner than later. Also, get any other vaccinations[18] you might need, so your Immune System can concentrate on fighting the Coronavirus and other day-to-day infections, stray pathogens, etc. Ask your Doctor what's right for you.

So what else can we do?

---

13. https://en.wikipedia.org/wiki/Misinformation_related_to_the_COVID-19_pandemic

14. https://en.wikipedia.org/wiki/List_of_unproven_methods_against_COVID-19

15. https://www.cdc.gov/coronavirus/2019-ncov/hcp/clinical-guidance-management-patients.html

16. https://www.who.int/emergencies/diseases/novel-coronavirus-2019/technical-guidance/patient-management

17. https://en.wikipedia.org/wiki/Influenza_vaccine

18. https://en.wikipedia.org/wiki/Vaccination_schedule

Beyond the treatments written above, I think more could be done to help a person recover and even to survive. Here's what I think could be done to help recovery/survival of CV, and most other illnesses for that matter...

Step 1 – Make Sure they "Want to Live"!

It's important to find out whether they Want to Live (Will to Live[19]). If so, why do they want to live? On the flip side, do they have perhaps a conscious or subconscious desire to die?

I think this is an important aspect to consider in any life-threatening medical situation. Doesn't this make sense? Why would you want to get better if there's nothing to live for? Some examples are below:

- Does a particular nursing home resident really want to go back to the nursing home with their life as it is there?
- Does a cancer patient really want to continue living in so much pain?
- If life before Coronavirus was so painful, why would someone want to get better and go back to that life?
- Has the person lost their zest for life and is just waiting to die?

The Will to Live is related to Quality of Life[20].

The Patient should be informed of the Potential Side Effects (Risks) of the proposed CV Treatment, as well as the Projected Outcomes (Benefits).

You, as a Doctor, and the Patient can decide whether it is better to do CV Treatment or just to let nature take its course, maybe even dying,

---

19. https://en.wikipedia.org/wiki/Will_to_live

20. https://en.wikipedia.org/wiki/Quality_of_life

if that's what happens... I think it's important to respect the Patient's Decision – whatever it is.

Step 2 - If the Patient is wanting and willing to do CV Treatment, then you could Maximize their "Motivation to Live" for best results.

To Find/Increase the "Motivation to Live" for the CV patient, consider the following.

- Get to know the CV Patient. Talk to them if you can. Talk with the family, friends, close others to find out what is/was important to the Patient.
- As a Doctor, if you are time/resource-limited, ask someone who does have the time and/or skill to do so, e.g. nurse, chaplain, family/friend, etc.
- What's important to them, e.g. religion, sports, family, work, etc.?
- Who is important in their lives, e.g. spouse, children, grandchildren, pets, etc.?
- Why would they like to continue living? Unfinished business? Unfulfilled dreams?
- Where would they like to go if they recover and what would they like to do? Do they have a "Bucket List"?
- When would they like to recover? Were they looking forward to an event before they got sick?
- How would they like to live once they get better? – i.e. a "New Lease on Life".
- In essence, find out what "Hope" means to them and encourage them to focus on that Hope instead of stressing out on how sick they are.
- Got Hope? – If not, try again to find some hope in the dying patient, otherwise, you might have to accept they just want to

die.

- The Will to Live is a giant component of Spontaneous Healing[21]. If interested, there is more information on Spontaneous Healing/Remission in this Chapter's References.

- In treatment, I think it is important to talk directly to the patient, even if they are not conscious. The patient might very well have some degree of awareness during anesthesia and might absorb your hopeful words/actions. I also think it is important to touch the patient if it is okay with the patient and/or others.

Step 3 – Suggest that Healing is going on even without a Real Vaccine.

- Maybe inform the Patient that the real work in combatting Coronavirus is our own Immune System. Vaccines[22] just "stimulates the body's immune system to recognize the agent as a threat, destroy it, and to further recognize and destroy any of the microorganisms associated with that agent that it may encounter in the future." Our Immune Systems do the "dirty work". Remind them to relax and just let their Immune System take care of the "nasty bug".
- Other powerful tools that are not used much in clinical practice are Hypnotherapy, Guided Imagery, and even Games. Some examples/clarifications are below.
  - Hypnosis is being used currently to unleash the Inner Healing Power in Patients who have Cancer and/or other Immune Disorders. Psychoneuroimmunology[23] uses many tools, one of

21. https://en.wikipedia.org/wiki/Spontaneous_remission

22. https://en.wikipedia.org/wiki/Vaccine

which is Hypnosis, e.g. Hypnotherapy and psychoneuroimmunology[24]. Some Coronavirus Hypnosis Scripts are becoming available, e.g. Hypnosis And Covid-19[25] .

○ Games are used with Cancer Patients to help them Imagine their Immune Systems Fighting Off Illness, e.g. Zapping Cancer Through Video Games[26]. Maybe someone will make a Zapping Game for the Coronavirus Bug, too, to at least get someone's mind off their condition, get them to relax, and maybe even trigger an internal immune response to the Coronavirus.

○ We're just beginning to learn about the Mind's Influence on our Immune Systems. Time will tell. What do we have to lose in using our Minds to Stimulate our own Internal Healing System? – even if we don't know exactly why or how it works. We have drugs with unknown "mechanisms of action",[27] yet we still use them. Why not use our Minds to help heal our Bodies? If it works, isn't it good?

Step 4 – Start "Positiveness/Hope Drip Therapy"

• <u>Whoever</u> goes into the patient's room, talk and act Positively. Remind the Patient of what they want to do when they get better. "Whoever" means doctors, nurses, lab techs, cleaning

---

23. https://en.wikipedia.org/wiki/Psychoneuroimmunology

24. https://www.hypnotherapy-directory.org.uk/memberarticles/hypnotherapy-and-psychoneuroimmunology

25. https://www.asch.net/Professionals/COVID.aspx

26. https://www.roswellpark.org/cancertalk/201307/zapping-cancer-through-video-games

27. https://en.wikipedia.org/wiki/Category:Drugs_with_unknown_mechanisms_of_action

personnel, etc. Speak even if you think the patient can't hear you.

- Doctors/Nurses – Be honest, but please say to the patient <u>any</u> progress at all. Even the hint of recovery inside a patient can work wonders. Watch your words and actions so that you don't trigger the Nocebo Effect[28]. Ask them if they see any signs of progress at all. Build on that. Encourage them to continue to relax and get better, reminding them their Immune System is working hard to combat any Coronavirus still left in their System.

- It's important to keep the patient quiet, calm, and relaxed so the Immune System is at full strength and not weakened by stress. I think I heard some hospitals, exercise places, etc. have blocked the News Stations from being selected by patients/patrons.

- Watch the words/actions of the Patient to detect and eliminate any Negative Stress. Listen to them. Look at their body language. Any Negative Stress is detrimental to the Immune System.

  - For now, all we have is words and body language to detect Stress/Pain. I predict someday, both Patients and Healthcare Workers will have Emotional Stress and/or Pain Monitors, probably wearable, like a wristband. Some years ago, I made a Medical Monitor with Emotional Stress Pain Indicator and Biofeedback[29] Prototype. It is very crude, yet I think it illustrates the potential of such a device.

- Give a periodic "Bolus" of Positiveness/Hope, e.g. hearing the voice of a grandchild saying "Please get better, Grandpa. Let's go fishing" – or the sound of a woodworking machine, if

---

28. https://en.wikipedia.org/wiki/Nocebo

29. https://www.youtube.com/watch?v=-r96IjiC6xg

their hobby is woodworking – or the sound of birds/frogs, if they are nature lovers – or anything at all that reminds them why they want to get better. Perhaps a slideshow of their favorite people, events, hopes, dreams, etc. might help too. All these are possible now even with social distancing/quarantining via technology. Again, please do this even if the patient does not seem to respond. You never know how a little thing can help a patient "turn the corner" toward recovery.

****

Don't give up communicating with Patients, even when they are unconscious and/or anesthetized. We're just starting to learn that listening and/or awareness goes on when we're unconscious, anesthetized, or even dying. Technology helps here with recordings, videos, maybe family members cheering on the Patient via electronic communication, e.g. Volunteers Are Collecting Tablets for COVID-19 Patients So They Don't Have to Suffer Alone[30].

****

All that being said, either the patient will get better or not.

- If they get better, thank yourself and the Universe. Be grateful.
- If they die, please know that you did your very best. It was just their time. Let it go.

Take-Aways

- With no Vaccine, Doctors and/or Patients might consider

---

30. https://time.com/5826220/covid-19-tablets/

Alternative Treatments, some of which are discussed in this Chapter.

- Psychoneuroimmunology[31] might relate to all the Steps above – making the patient relaxed, motivating their will to live, and soaking them in an atmosphere of positivity and hope.
- Maybe trying "something" is better than doing nothing, as long as it is safe. Doctors can look at the big picture of whether a particular "something" is safe and would be beneficial for a particular patient.
- *Patients - It is very important that you check with your doctor to see if the "something" you found is right for you.*

Reminder for Patients – Continue following Local and/or Personalized CV Prevention Guidelines until your Doctor says it is safe to lessen or discontinue them. Please get the Coronavirus Vaccine when it becomes available and is reliable – trust your doctor to help you decide what is right for you. In addition, please get annual flu shots[32] and any other vaccinations your doctor might think is right for you, e.g. Pneumonia Vaccine[33], etc.

Jump to this Chapters References or otherwise keep reading to go to the next chapter.

31. https://en.wikipedia.org/wiki/Psychoneuroimmunology

32. https://en.wikipedia.org/wiki/Influenza_vaccine

33. https://en.wikipedia.org/wiki/Pneumococcal_vaccine

Chapter 5 – Conclusion

Wow, did we cover a lot of ground in this book...Let's unponder all that we've done...

- We looked at Coronavirus from the Outside-In and the Inside-Out (Chapter 1).
- In Chapter 2, we delved into what all affects our Immune System. We learned how to Boost/Maintain our Immune System to Maximum "Fighting Strength" - to ward off Coronaviruses as well as other Nasties.
- In Chapter 3, we learned what we could do personally to help ourselves and maybe others, especially our children.

- Chapter 4 is what your doctor could do to help you get better and stay better. If you see something you like, talk it over with your doctor to see if it is right for you.

Before you finish this book, be sure to check out the Appendix that shows...

- References for each Chapter;
- Search Strings to find more References like those provided;
- Contact Information.

We all have been affected by this Pandemic, in one way or another. Some of us might have been diagnosed with Coronavirus – this is a physical diagnosis. From what I see and hear most, if not all of us, are trying to cope with the psychological and emotional aspect of this pandemic, though. Time will tell how this pandemic will linger on in our lives physically, mentally, and maybe even spiritually as the days, weeks, months, and years go on. This book might at least give you some ideas and/or resources for now and in the future, if needed.

Jump to the Appendix - Chapter References, Search Strings, Other Useful Information or otherwise keep reading to go to the Epilogue.

Epilogue

I hope you found this book helpful. I did.

It really helped me to get my thoughts and feelings out on paper – to write about them. As I was writing, I was thinking that my efforts might help someone, which made me feel good. In addition, researching and writing kept my mind busy during troubling times. Now, with this book done, I have to find something else to stay mentally active, healthy, and hopefully helpful. Stay tuned, if interested.

I wish you all well - and hope you all "get better" and "stay better". ☺

Tom Garz

The End (of this book)

Appendix - Chapter References, Search Strings, Other Useful Information

CHAPTER REFERENCES are below...

Jump to **SEARCH STRINGS**

Jump to **CONTACT ME**

****

CHAPTER REFERENCES for Each Chapter...

Please note that the References below are just a Snapshot in Time. Some references might apply to more than one chapter. Use Search Strings in this Appendix to "Find More Like These".

****

REFERENCES for Chapter 1 – Coronavirus - The Inside Story

2020 coronavirus pandemic in the United States[1]

'A Ruffled Mind Makes A Restless Pillow': Bad Dreams, Disturbed Sleep And The Coronavirus[2]

Anxiety and the coronavirus pandemic[3]

Colorado schools sound the alarm on students' emotional well-being during coronavirus crisis[4]

---

1. https://en.wikipedia.org/wiki/2020_coronavirus_pandemic_in_the_United_States

2. https://www.wbur.org/hereandnow/2020/04/23/coronavirus-sleep-dreams

3. https://www.myjoyonline.com/lifestyle/anxiety-and-the-coronavirus-pandemic/

4. https://coloradosun.com/2020/04/20/colorado-schools-coronavirus-mental-health/

Common Human Coronaviruses[5]

Compassion fatigue and burnout in nursing : enhancing professional quality of life[6]

Coronavirus[7]

Coronavirus[8]

Coronavirus — COVID-19[9]

Coronavirus disease[10]

Coronavirus Disease (COVID-19): Psychological, Behavioral, Interpersonal Effects, and Clinical Implications for Health Systems[11]

Coronavirus disease 2019[12]

CSIRO study reveals negative impact of COVID-19 on weight and emotional wellbeing[13]

Dedicated Workers[14]

---

5. https://www.cdc.gov/coronavirus/
   general-information.html?fbclid=IwAR2bL4iB84iqmbyTwwoQSVoKjxZasKFuCf_1TzKQNAs
   aPjobTI57Jgc0LXY

6. http://www.worldcat.org/oclc/1060577411

7. https://en.wikipedia.org/wiki/Coronavirus_disease_2019

8. https://hesperian.org/2020/03/05/coronavirus/

9. https://en.hesperian.org/hhg/Coronavirus

10. https://en.wikipedia.org/wiki/Coronavirus_disease_2019

11. https://www.frontiersin.org/research-topics/13561/
    coronavirus-disease-covid-19-psychological-behavioral-interpersonal-effects-and-clinical-implica
    tion

12. https://en.wikipedia.org/wiki/Coronavirus_disease_2019

13. https://www.news-medical.net/news/20200617/
    CSIRO-study-reveals-negative-impact-of-COVID-19-on-weight-and-emotional-wellbeing.aspx

Depression can't hit a moving target' | The mental health pattern impacting San Diegans during the pandemic[15]

Feeling drained by coronavirus quarantine? Science can explain why[16]

Half Of Americans Suffering Mental Health Issues During Coronavirus, New Poll Shows[17]

Having weird dreams in quarantine? You're not alone.[18]

How the coronavirus pandemic is infiltrating our subconscious, affecting dreams[19]

'i dream of covid' Tracks Subconscious Under Quarantine[20]

Is returning to work during the COVID-19 pandemic stressful? A study on immediate mental health status and psychoneuroimmunity prevention measures of Chinese workforce[21]

---

14. https://www.thehitavada.com/Encyc/2020/4/29/Dedicated-Workers.html

15. https://www.cbs8.com/article/news/health/
    depression-cant-hit-a-moving-target-the-mental-health-pattern-impacting-san-diegans-during-t
    he-pandemic/509-a7bc8324-c6e7-4986-b344-aef6ca2b8ebd

16. https://www.latimes.com/science/story/2020-04-29/
    what-science-tells-us-about-the-psychological-impacts-of-coronavirus-isolation

17. https://www.forbes.com/sites/geekgirlrising/2020/04/06/
    half-of-americans-say-covid-19-is-hurting-their-mental-health-new-poll-shows/#bba22c5351e3

18. https://www.vox.com/the-goods/2020/4/9/21215312/
    quarantine-vivid-dreams-psychologist-q-and-a

19. https://www.thedenverchannel.com/news/local-news/
    how-the-coronavirus-pandemic-is-infiltrating-our-subconscious-affecting-dreams

20. https://www.npr.org/2020/04/13/833623332/
    i-dream-of-covid-tracks-subconscious-under-quarantine?utm_medium=RSS&utm_campaign=
    artslife

21. https://www.ncbi.nlm.nih.gov/pmc/articles/PMC7179503/

Mental health and psychosocial considerations during the COVID-19 outbreak - WHO[22]

New research links supernatural causal beliefs about COVID-19 to clinical emotional problems[23]

New study shows Australians suffering weight gain and emotional hardship due to coronavirus pandemic[24]

Opinion: COVID-19 is also a subconscious epidemic[25]

Our pandemic subconscious: why we seem to be dreaming much more – and often of insects - Stress can affect the quality and length of sleep. Scientists have been collecting dream data during the coronavirus crisis, with surprising results[26]

People in coronavirus quarantine are comfort eating and this has nutritionists worried about obesity levels[27]

People tune out facts and trust their guts in medical emergencies[28]

---

22. https://www.who.int/docs/default-source/coronaviruse/mental-health-considerations.pdf

23. https://www.psypost.org/2020/06/
    new-research-links-supernatural-causal-beliefs-about-covid-19-to-clinical-emotional-problems-5
    6989

24. https://www.9news.com.au/national/
    csiro-study-find-australians-gaining-weight-suffering-decline-emotional-wellbeing-during-coron
    avirus-lockdown/6a1d71c8-5df3-4d1e-8eaa-778aa9436301

25. https://universitystar.com/36566/opinions/opinion-covid-19-is-also-a-subconscious-epidemic/

26. https://www.theguardian.com/lifeandstyle/2020/apr/30/
    our-pandemic-subconscious-why-we-seem-to-be-dreaming-much-more-and-often-of-insects

27. https://www.msn.com/en-au/news/australia/
    people-in-coronavirus-quarantine-are-comfort-eating-and-this-has-nutritionists-worried-about-
    obesity-levels/ar-BB12ugAT

28. https://www.sciencedaily.com/releases/2020/04/200403131259.htm

Physiological Data Collected from Wearable AI-Powered Technology Reveals Negative Emotions Have Almost Doubled Since Lockdown - A breakthrough in the mental health industry as the Feel Program quantifies COVID-19's Impact on Our Mental Health for the First Time[29]

Robert Emmons: Science anxiety in the time of Covid[30]

Severe acute respiratory syndrome coronavirus 2[31]

Social determinants of health[32]

The Cultural Psychology of the COVID-19 Pandemic[33]

The hidden struggle: The mental health effects of the Covid-19 lockdown in South Africa[34]

The Impact Of Early Life Trauma On Health And Disease : The Hidden Epidemic[35]

The pandemic is giving people vivid, unusual dreams. Here's why.[36]

29. https://www.businesswire.com/news/home/20200507005691/en/
   Physiological-Data-Collected-Wearable-AI-Powered-Technology-Reveals

30. https://vtdigger.org/2020/06/09/robert-emmons-science-anxiety-in-the-time-of-covid/

31. https://en.wikipedia.org/wiki/Severe_acute_respiratory_syndrome_coronavirus_2

32. https://en.wikipedia.org/wiki/Social_determinants_of_health

33. https://www.frontiersin.org/research-topics/14544/
   the-cultural-psychology-of-the-covid-19-pandemic?fbclid=IwAR1KBtDsjzzBuSu3uT_piDJx9ig
   T6ID_kWVsSgOFADEhWx3nILaf6zUPXyU

34. https://www.dailymaverick.co.za/article/
   2020-05-13-the-hidden-struggle-the-mental-health-effects-of-the-covid-19-lockdown-in-south-a
   frica/

35. http://www.worldcat.org/oclc/874670449

36. https://www.nationalgeographic.com/science/2020/04/
   coronavirus-pandemic-is-giving-people-vivid-unusual-dreams-here-is-why/

The Psychology of Pandemics[37]

Unintended Consequences of CoVid-19[38]

Why is lockdown such an emotional rollercoaster? Experts tell us what is happening with your brain, and your children, and why it's not always good to 'stay positive'[39]

Why your dreams are so vivid in lockdown[40]

Coronavirus impacts BAME children's mental health more than white peers, research shows[41]

JUMP BACK TO Chapter 2 – Let's Keep Our Immune System Happy and Healthy

****

REFERENCES for Chapter 2 – Let's Keep Our Immune System Happy and Healthy

5. Health determinants[42]

6 Signs You Have a Weakened Immune System[43]

---

37. https://www.google.com/books/edition/The_Psychology_of_Pandemics/
    YrWryQEACAAJ?hl=en

38. https://www.baylor.edu/medical_humanities/doc.php/353378.pdf

39. https://www.manchestereveningnews.co.uk/news/greater-manchester-news/
    lockdown-emotional-rollercoaster-experts-tell-18133695

40. https://www.culturewhisper.com/r/lifestyle/
    why_are_my_dreams_so_vivid_in_lockdown_dreams_meaning/15641

41. https://www.cypnow.co.uk/news/article/
    coronavirus-impacts-bame-children-s-mental-health-more-than-white-peers-research-shows

42. https://www.who.int/bulletin/africanhealth2014/health_determinants/en/

An Elegant Defense: The Extraordinary New Science of the Immune System: A Tale in Four Lives[44]

Consumption of liquor can weaken immunity, increase chances of COVID-19 infection[45]

COVID-19 infection: the perspectives on immune responses[46]

Diet and Immune Function[47]

Diet and Your Immune System: A COVID-19 Related Update[48]

Diet Can Fight Diseases Linked to Poor COVID-19 Outcomes[49]

Eat more fruits and vegetables to improve your immune system. Five or more portions of fruits and vegetables daily significantly increase antibody response.[50]

Eating during COVID-19: Improve your mood and lower stress[51]

---

43. https://www.pennmedicine.org/updates/blogs/health-and-wellness/2020/march/
weakened-immune-system

44. https://books.google.com/
books?id=pLRnDwAAQBAJ&newbks=1&newbks_redir=0&dq=(%22coronavirus%22+OR
+%22covid%22+OR+%E2%80%9Ccovida%E2%80%9D)+%E2%80%9Cimmune+system%E
2%80%9D&source=gbs_navlinks_s

45. https://newslivetv.com/
consumption-of-liquor-can-weaken-immunity-increase-chances-of-covid-19-infection/

46. https://www.nature.com/articles/s41418-020-0530-3

47. https://www.ncbi.nlm.nih.gov/pmc/articles/PMC6723551/

48. https://www.krh.org/news/diet-and-your-immune-system-a-covid-19-related-update/

49. https://www.pcrm.org/news/blog/diet-can-fight-diseases-linked-poor-covid-19-outcomes

50. https://www.ncbi.nlm.nih.gov/pubmed/23495421

51. https://www.health.harvard.edu/blog/
eating-during-covid-19-improve-your-mood-and-lower-stress-2020040719409

Effects of air pollutants on innate immunity: The role of Toll-like receptors and nucleotide-binding oligomerization domain–like receptors[52]

Effects of stress on immune cell distribution. Dynamics and hormonal mechanisms[53]

Enkephalins and Endorphins: Stress and the Immune System[54]

Environmental Influences on the Immune System[55]

Exercise boosts immune response.[56]

Exercise, Immunity and the COVID-19 Pandemic[57]

Feeding the immune system.[58]

Fighting an illness? 4 ways to boost your immune system[59]

Fight-or-flight response[60]

---

52. https://www.ncbi.nlm.nih.gov/pmc/articles/PMC4341993/

53. https://www.ncbi.nlm.nih.gov/pubmed/7730652

54. https://books.google.com/
    books?id=4Gn1BwAAQBAJ&newbks=1&newbks_redir=0&dq=%22immune+system%E2%80%9D+(psychological+OR+emotional+OR+%22mental+health%22)&source=gbs_navlinks_s

55. https://books.google.com/
    books?id=-T6FCwAAQBAJ&newbks=1&newbks_redir=0&dq=(%22coronavirus%22+OR+%22covid%22+OR+%E2%80%9Ccovida%E2%80%9D)+%E2%80%9Cimmune+system%E2%80%9D&source=gbs_navlinks_s

56. https://www.ncbi.nlm.nih.gov/pubmed/27750511

57. https://www.acsm.org/blog-detail/acsm-blog/2020/03/30/
    exercise-immunity-covid-19-pandemic

58. https://www.ncbi.nlm.nih.gov/pubmed/23688939

59. https://www.lls.org/blog/fighting-an-illness-4-ways-to-boost-your-immune-system

Foods and drinks that compromise your immune system[61]

Handbook of human stress and immunity[62]

Handbook of personality and health[63]

Handbook of religion and health[64]

Handbook of religion and mental health[65]

Healing and the Mind: Emotions and the Immune System[66]

Herd immunity[67]

Here's Why You Should Be Drinking Plenty Of Water During The Coronavirus Lockdown[68]

How Sleep Affects Your Immunity[69]

How stress and loneliness can make you more likely to get COVID-19[70]

---

60. https://en.wikipedia.org/wiki/Fight-or-flight_response

61. https://www.piedmont.org/living-better/
    foods-and-drinks-that-compromise-your-immune-system

62. http://www.worldcat.org/oclc/248410692

63. http://www.worldcat.org/oclc/845529973

64. http://www.worldcat.org/oclc/1029102381

65. http://www.worldcat.org/oclc/838061039

66. https://www.simmsmanncenter.ucla.edu/center_events/
    healing-and-the-mind-emotions-and-the-immune-system/

67. https://en.wikipedia.org/wiki/Herd_immunity

68. https://www.forbes.com/sites/daviddisalvo/2020/03/22/
    heres-why-you-should-be-drinking-plenty-of-water-during-the-coronavirus-lockdown/#a5c0239
    3e59c943d6a75a9241140faca317f086363f47

69. https://www.sleepfoundation.org/articles/how-sleep-affects-your-immunity

How stress damages immune system and health.[71]

How Stress Helps The Immune System[72]

How the Immune System Works[73]

How to boost your immune system[74]

How to boost your immune system to avoid colds and coronavirus[75]

How To Boost Your Immunity To Stay Healthy[76]

How To Strengthen Your Immune System With The Power Of Your Mind[77]

I'm Immune! How Your Immune System Keeps You Safe - Health Books for Kids - Children's Disease Books[78]

---

70. https://news.rice.edu/2020/03/19/
    how-stress-and-loneliness-can-make-you-more-likely-to-get-covid-19/

71. https://www.ncbi.nlm.nih.gov/pubmed/20704904

72. https://www.medicalnewstoday.com/articles/247216.php

73. https://books.google.com/
    books?id=Vb-SCgAAQBAJ&newbks=1&newbks_redir=0&dq=(%22coronavirus%22+OR+
    %22covid%22+OR+%E2%80%9Ccovida%E2%80%9D)+%E2%80%9Cimmune+system%E2
    %80%9D&source=gbs_navlinks_s

74. https://www.health.harvard.edu/staying-healthy/how-to-boost-your-immune-system

75. https://www.theguardian.com/lifeandstyle/2020/mar/08/
    how-to-boost-your-immune-system-to-avoid-colds-and-coronavirus

76. https://www.femina.in/wellness/how-to-boost-your-immunity-to-stay-healthy-154424.html

77. https://www.yourtango.com/experts/caroline-rushforth/
    how-strengthen-your-immune-system-with-your-mind

78. https://books.google.com/
    books?id=wYsFMQAACAAJ&dq=(%22coronavirus%22+OR+%22covid%22+OR+%E2%80
    %9Ccovida%E2%80%9D)+%E2%80%9Cimmune+system%E2%80%9D&hl=en&newbks=1

Immune cycle[79]

Immune system[80]

Immunodeficiency[81]

Impact of Nutrition and Diet on COVID-19 Infection and Implications for Kidney Health and Kidney Disease Management.[82]

Links between coronavirus, nutrition and the immune system[83]

Mind-Body Medicine and Immune System Outcomes: A Systematic Review[84]

Neural-immune interactions in health and disease[85]

Neurobiology of the Immune System[86]

Nutritional and Physical Activity Interventions to Improve Immunity[87]

&newbks_redir=0&sa=X&ved=2ahUKEwiWue7m9N7oAhXPK80KHSWmDKs4UBDoAT AAegQIABAC

79. https://en.wikipedia.org/wiki/Immune_cycle

80. https://en.wikipedia.org/wiki/Immune_system

81. https://en.wikipedia.org/wiki/Immunodeficiency

82. https://www.ncbi.nlm.nih.gov/pubmed/32291198

83. https://www.wcrf.org/int/blog/articles/2020/04/
links-between-coronavirus-nutrition-and-immune-system

84. https://www.ncbi.nlm.nih.gov/pmc/articles/PMC3516431/

85. https://www.ncbi.nlm.nih.gov/pubmed/12114255

86. https://books.google.com/
books?id=FuoGdGCB1j0C&newbks=1&newbks_redir=0&dq=%22immune+system%E2%8 0%9D+(psychological+OR+emotional+OR+%22mental+health%22)&source=gbs_navlinks_ s

87. https://www.ncbi.nlm.nih.gov/pmc/articles/PMC6124954/

---

88. https://journals.sagepub.com/doi/abs/10.1111/j.0963-7214.2005.00345.x?journalCode=cdpa

89. https://books2read.com/u/mBgJnA

90. https://www.ncbi.nlm.nih.gov/pmc/articles/PMC5681483/

91. https://www.ncbi.nlm.nih.gov/pmc/articles/PMC1361287/

92. https://kilthub.cmu.edu/articles/Psychological_Stress_Immunity_and_Physical_Disease/5099050/1

93. https://socialwork.buffalo.edu/content/dam/socialwork/home/self-care-kit/exercises/strengthen-your-immune-system.pdf

94. https://www.apa.org/news/press/releases/2004/07/stress-immune

95. https://books.google.com/books?id=q2CRDwAAQBAJ&newbks=1&newbks_redir=0&dq=%22immune+system%E2%80%9D+(psychological+OR+emotional+OR+%22mental+health%22)&source=gbs_navlinks_s

Stress Weakens the Immune System[97]

Stress, Age, and Immune Function: Toward a Lifespan Approach[98]

Stress, depression and the activation of the immune system.[99]

Stress, immune reactivity and susceptibility to infectious disease[100]

Stress, Inflammation, Immunity[101]

Stress, Personal Relationships, and Immune Function: Health Implications[102]

Stress-associated immune dysregulation and its importance for human health: a personal history of psychoneuroimmunology.[103]

Stressor-Induced Alterations of Adaptive Immunity to Vaccination and Viral Pathogens[104]

Stress-related disorders[105]

Super Immunity: The Essential Nutrition Guide for Boosting Your Body's Defenses to Live Longer, Stronger, and Disease Free[106]

96. https://www.ncbi.nlm.nih.gov/pubmed/2568569

97. https://www.apa.org/research/action/immune

98. https://www.ncbi.nlm.nih.gov/pmc/articles/PMC2805089/

99. https://www.ncbi.nlm.nih.gov/pubmed/12607229

100. https://www.cmu.edu/dietrich/psychology/stress-immunity-disease-lab/abstracts/pdf/ marslandbachen02.pdf

101. https://www.rn.com/featured-stories/stress-inflammation-immunity/

102. https://pdfs.semanticscholar.org/57b4/c04d60b2c902ebf9fefe24432821cae8ef83.pdf

103. https://www.ncbi.nlm.nih.gov/pubmed/15581732

104. https://www.ncbi.nlm.nih.gov/pmc/articles/PMC3339561/

105. https://en.wikipedia.org/wiki/Stress-related_disorders

106. https://books.google.com/ books?id=a9-QeXEmN9EC&newbks=1&newbks_redir=0&dq=(%22coronavirus%22+OR+

Support a Healthy Immune System with P3[107]

The 30-Minute Immune System Diet Plan: Quick Recipes to Strengthen Immunity and Prevent Disease[108]

The Immune Response: Basic and Clinical Principles[109]

The Immune System and Mental Health[110]

The Immune System Cure: Optimize Your Immune System in 30 Days-The Natural Way![111]

The Immune System Recovery Plan: A Doctor's 4-Step Program to Treat Autoimmune Disease[112]

%22covid%22+OR+%E2%80%9Ccovida%E2%80%9D)+%E2%80%9Cimmune+system%E2%80%9D&source=gbs_navlinks_s

107. https://p3.amedd.army.mil/trending-topics/support-a-healthy-immune-system-with-p3

108. https://books.google.com/
books?id=S-DlxwEACAAJ&dq=(%22coronavirus%22+OR+%22covid%22+OR+%E2%80%9Ccovida%E2%80%9D)+%E2%80%9Cimmune+system%E2%80%9D&hl=en&newbks=1&newbks_redir=0&sa=X&ved=2ahUKEwih7Yy-9N7oAhUGOs0KHenVBBU4RhDoATAEegQIABAB

109. https://books.google.com/
books?id=2AaJqNl1QIYC&newbks=1&newbks_redir=0&dq=(%22coronavirus%22+OR+%22covid%22+OR+%E2%80%9Ccovida%E2%80%9D)+%E2%80%9Cimmune+system%E2%80%80%9D&source=gbs_navlinks_s

110. https://books.google.com/
books?id=wqNPDwAAQBAJ&newbks=1&newbks_redir=0&dq=%22immune+system%E2%80%9D+(psychological+OR+emotional+OR+%22mental+health%22)&source=gbs_navlinks_s

111. https://books.google.com/
books?id=EDajgKKO1woC&newbks=1&newbks_redir=0&dq=%22immune+system%E2%80%9D+(psychological+OR+emotional+OR+%22mental+health%22)&source=gbs_navlinks_s

JUMP BACK TO Chapter 3 – So, What Can We Do About It?

****

REFERENCES for Chapter 3 – So, What Can We Do About It?

112. https://books.google.com/
   books?id=PE6K_PRO1RAC&newbks=1&newbks_redir=0&dq=(%22coronavirus%22+OR+%22covid%22+OR+%E2%80%9Ccovida%E2%80%9D)+%E2%80%9Cimmune+system%E2%80%9D&source=gbs_navlinks_s

113. https://www.ncbi.nlm.nih.gov/pmc/articles/PMC7165103/

114. https://health.clevelandclinic.org/what-happens-when-your-immune-system-gets-stressed-out/

115. https://books.google.com/
   books?id=BBWorCaG_zUC&newbks=1&newbks_redir=0&dq=%22immune+system%E2%80%9D+(psychological+OR+emotional+OR+%22mental+health%22)&source=gbs_navlinks_s

116. https://thriveglobal.com/stories/
   first-responders-coronavirus-reframe-anxiety-stress-management-tips/

117. https://www.who.int/news-room/campaigns/connecting-the-world-to-combat-Coronavirus/
   healthyathome/
   healthyathome---mental-health?gclid=EAIaIQobChMIiNaMtr6s6QIVjf7jBx34MwsLEAMYA
   SAAEgI2BvD_BwE

"moodgym[118] is like an interactive self-help book which helps you to learn and practise skills which can help to prevent and manage symptoms of depression and anxiety."

<u>100 things to do while stuck inside due to a pandemic[119]</u>

<u>100 useful things you can do to kill boredom if you're quarantined at home because of coronavirus[120]</u>

<u>100+ Fun Things to Do at Home Right Now, From Virtual Tours to Animals Cams and More[121]</u>

<u>5 Ways Seniors Can Stay Active During COVID-19 Social Distancing[122]</u>

<u>5 Ways to Boost Your Immune System[123]</u>

<u>50 Fun Things You Can Do at Home Right Now in Quarantine[124]</u>

<u>50 things to do while you're stuck inside during quarantine[125]</u>

<u>6 books a psychologist says can free you from anxiety and stress[126]</u>

---

118. https://moodgym.com.au/

119. https://www.usatoday.com/story/life/health-wellness/2020/03/16/
     coronavirus-quarantine-100-things-do-while-trapped-inside/5054632002/

120. https://i-d.vice.com/en_uk/article/n7jk77/
     100-things-to-do-quarantine-home-coronavirus-self-isolation-social-distancing

121. https://www.travelandleisure.com/travel-tips/
     fun-things-to-do-at-home-during-coronavirus-quarantine

122. https://www.visitingangels.com/knowledge-center/senior-health-and-well-being/
     5-ways-seniors-can-stay-active-during-covid-19-social-distancing/499

123. https://www.aarp.org/health/healthy-living/info-2020/boosting-immune-response.html

124. https://www.thrillist.com/news/nation/things-to-do-in-quarantine-fun-ideas-bored-at-home

125. https://www.dailycal.org/2020/04/03/
     50-things-to-do-while-youre-stuck-inside-during-quarantine/

126. https://www.businessinsider.sg/

   psychologist-books-free-anxiety-stress-coronavirus-social-distancing-grief-2020-4

127. https://www.cnet.com/health/

   7-things-to-not-do-when-coronavirus-lockdown-and-quarantine-end/

128. https://www.ncoa.org/blog/

   7-tips-for-managing-your-mental-health-during-the-covid-19-pandemic/?dxk=H4sIAAAAAA

   AEAKtWKs4vLUpOVbJScs1LT0xPVdJRSk7MLUjMTM8DimXmZZZkJpZklqUWx-gbGhtY

   GirVAgBz2_UiMwAAAA2

129. https://www.hackensackmeridianhealth.org/HealthU/2020/05/07/

   7-ways-to-stimulate-brain-health-during-a-lockdown/

130. https://www.letssaythanks.com/

   brain-games-for-seniors/?dxk=H4sIAAAAAAAEAKtWKs4vLUpOVbJScs1LT0xPVdJRSk7M

   LUjMTM8DimXmZZZkJpZklqUWx-gbGhtYGijVAgBEsTcjMwAAAA2

131. https://www.forbes.com/sites/williamarruda/2020/03/15/

   9-ways-to-stay-positive-during-the-coronavirus-pandemic/#a5c02393e59c943d6a75a9241140fa

   ca3268508da5a8e

132. https://www.eurekalert.org/pub_releases/2020-04/bu-9rr043020.php

A List Of Live Virtual Concerts To Watch During The Coronavirus Shutdown[134]

A Systems Approach to Stress, Stressors and Resilience in Humans[135]

Americans' COVID-19 Stress, Coping, and Adherence to CDC Guidelines.[136]

Amidst COVID-19, Black psychologist, others tell African Americans how to maintain mental, emotional health[137]

Anxious Jaxon - A Brand New World: A coping tale for Covid-19[138]

APA COVID-19 Information and Resources[139] - American Psychological Association.

Beck Depression Inventory[140]

Become Aware of Your Stressors and Reactions[141]

133. http://www.worldcat.org/oclc/8587364136

134. https://www.npr.org/2020/03/17/816504058/
a-list-of-live-virtual-concerts-to-watch-during-the-coronavirus-shutdown?dxk=H4sIAAAAAA
AEAKtWKs4vLUpOVbJScs1LT0xPVdJRSk7MLUjMTM8DimXmZZZkJpZklqUWx-gbGhtY
GijVAgBEsTcjMwAAAA2

135. https://www.ncbi.nlm.nih.gov/pmc/articles/PMC4323923/

136. http://www.worldcat.org/oclc/8602145888

137. http://www.louisianaweekly.com/
amidst-covid-19-black-psychologist-others-tell-african-americans-how-to-maintain-mental-emot
ional-health/

138. https://www.amazon.com/Anxious-Jaxon-Brand-coping-Covid-19-ebook/dp/
B086VQTWQD/
ref=sr_1_7?dchild=1&keywords=%28%22coronavirus%22+%22covid%22+%28coping&qid=
1586555419&sr=8-7

139. http://www.worldcat.org/oclc/1149151453

140. https://en.wikipedia.org/wiki/Beck_Depression_Inventory

141. https://www.takingcharge.csh.umn.edu/enhance-your-wellbeing/health/stress-mastery/become-aware-your-stressors-and-reactions

142. https://www.ncbi.nlm.nih.gov/pmc/articles/PMC3893969/

143. http://citeseerx.ist.psu.edu/viewdoc/download?doi=10.1.1.300.4923&rep=rep1&type=pdf

144. https://www.djournal.com/opinion/bill-crawford-help-others-cope-with-pandemic-fear-and-anxiety/article_99645ed0-ac16-56d3-aeb9-a98feb5048fc.html

145. https://www.srqmagazine.com/srq-daily/2020-04-13/13236_Brain+Health+Boost+from+Music

146. https://theconversation.com/brain-research-shows-the-arts-promote-mental-health-136668

147. http://www.worldcat.org/oclc/930853037

148. https://www.cdc.gov/coronavirus/2019-ncov/community/index.html

149. https://www.theeagle.com/news/health_fitness/c-force-we-all-must-soldier-on-in-the-covid-19-era/article_9cb63530-9e12-11ea-8c0b-e766fabb9f13.html

150. https://starr.org/

      childrens-mental-health-awareness-in-times-of-covid-19/?utm_source=mailchimp&utm_mediu
      m=email&utm_content=button&utm_campaign=may2020week2

151. https://thriveglobal.com/stories/

      close-relationships-can-buffer-the-negative-effects-of-stress-in-a-crisis/

152. http://www.worldcat.org/oclc/1150888399

153. https://www.amazon.com/Coping-During-Pandemic-Self-exploration-Journal/dp/
      B086G1XSR1/

      ref=sr_1_24?dchild=1&keywords=%28%22coronavirus%22+%22covid%22+%28coping&qid
      =1586555638&sr=8-24

154. https://www.amazon.com/Coping-National-Crisis-Journal-Family/dp/B086PTFQYT/

      ref=sr_1_20?dchild=1&keywords=%28%22coronavirus%22+%22covid%22+%28coping&qid
      =1586555910&sr=8-20

155. https://www.amazon.com/Coping-Confinement-During-COVID-19-Couples-ebook/dp/
      B086T68ZR9/

      ref=sr_1_4?dchild=1&keywords=%28%22coronavirus%22+%22covid%22+%28coping&qid=
      1586555365&sr=8-4

156. https://books.google.com/

      books?id=bhTYDwAAQBAJ&printsec=frontcover&dq=Coping+with+Coronavirus:+How+

Corona means no face touching. Science shows we can't help it[157]

Coronavirus and its Nocebo effect: Here is what it means and why you should avoid it at all costs[158]

Coronavirus lockdown: fresh data on compliance and public opinion[159]

Coronavirus Vs Books: Reading Books For Surviving Home During A Pandemic. Advices On 20 Timeless Masterpieces To Spend Time And Find Peace Of Mind During Covid-19 Quarantine[160]

---

to+Stay+Calm+and+Protect+your+Mental+Health&hl=en&newbks=1&newbks_redir=0&s

a=X&ved=2ahUKEwict57A6t7oAhUWXM0KHfO6CjUQ6AEwAHoECAQQAg#v_43ec3e

5dee6e706af7766fffea512721_onepage_6cff047854f19ac2aa52aac51bf3af4a_q_43ec3e5dee6e

706af7766fffea512721_Coping_0bcef9c45bd8a48eda1b26eb0c61c869_20with_0bcef9c45bd8

a48eda1b26eb0c61c869_20Coronavirus_0bcef9c45bd8a48eda1b26eb0c61c869_3A_0bcef9c4

5bd8a48eda1b26eb0c61c869_20How_0bcef9c45bd8a48eda1b26eb0c61c869_20to_0bcef9c4

5bd8a48eda1b26eb0c61c869_20Stay_0bcef9c45bd8a48eda1b26eb0c61c869_20Calm_0bcef9

c45bd8a48eda1b26eb0c61c869_20and_0bcef9c45bd8a48eda1b26eb0c61c869_20Protect_0bc

ef9c45bd8a48eda1b26eb0c61c869_20your_0bcef9c45bd8a48eda1b26eb0c61c869_20Mental_

0bcef9c45bd8a48eda1b26eb0c61c869_20Health_6cff047854f19ac2aa52aac51bf3af4a_f_43ec

3e5dee6e706af7766fffea512721_false

157. https://jewishstandard.timesofisrael.com/

corona-means-no-face-touching-science-shows-we-cant-help-it/

158. https://timesofindia.indiatimes.com/life-style/health-fitness/health-news/

coronavirus-and-its-nocebo-effect-here-is-what-it-means-and-why-you-should-avoid-it-at-all-cos

ts/articleshow/74622955.cms

159. https://theconversation.com/

coronavirus-lockdown-fresh-data-on-compliance-and-public-opinion-135872

160. https://www.amazon.com/

CORONAVIRUS-BOOKS-SURVIVING-MASTERPIECES-QUARANTINE-ebook/dp/

B086T1GHZH/

ref=sr_1_fkmr0_2?dchild=1&keywords=%28%22coronavirus%22+OR+%22covid%22+OR+

Coronavirus: 10 sports books to beat the lockdown blues[161]

Coronavirus: how to manage stress eating during self-isolation[162]

Coronavirus: Mental Health Coping Strategies[163]

COVID - 19 Everything will be fine: How to overcome the emergency by staying at home[164]

COVID-19 lockdown: Be mindful of the emotional health of your kids[165]

COVID-19 Resource and Information Guide[166]

Covid-19 Strategy Update[167]

Covid-19 Stress and Coping - CDC[168]

COVID-19 survivor, father of 3, speaks about his 'mental journey' after fighting virus[169]

%E2%80%9Ccovida%E2%80%9D%29+%28coping+OR+psychological+OR+emotional+OR +%22mental+health%22%29&qid=1586555309&sr=8-2-fkmr0

161. https://sportstar.thehindu.com/other-sports/ coronavirus-ten-classic-sports-books-to-read-during-covid-19-lockdown-extension-gavaskar-bra dman-muhammad-ali-olympics-reading-list-cricket-boxing/article31321630.ece

162. https://www.netdoctor.co.uk/healthy-eating/a32081695/stress-eating/

163. https://www.nami.org/Blogs/NAMI-Blog/March-2020/ Coronavirus-Mental-Health-Coping-Strategies

164. https://www.google.com/books/edition/COVID_19_Everything_will_be_fine/ FP_ZDwAAQBAJ?hl=en&gbpv=0

165. https://www.expresshealthcare.in/blogs/ covid-19-lockdown-be-mindful-of-the-emotional-health-of-your-kids/420886/

166. https://www.nami.org/covid-19-guide

167. https://www.who.int/docs/default-source/coronaviruse/covid-strategy-update-14april2020.pdf

168. https://www.cdc.gov/coronavirus/2019-ncov/daily-life-coping/managing-stress-anxiety.html

---

169. https://wjla.com/news/coronavirus/survivor-speaks-of-mental-journey-after-beating-covid-19

170. https://www.kitchenertoday.com/coronavirus-covid-19-national-news/
covid-19-the-surprising-reasons-people-cheat-at-social-distancing-2377833

171. https://www.amazon.com/COVID-19-THIS-TOO-SHALL-PASS-ebook/dp/
B086CFB1XT/
ref=sr_1_13?dchild=1&keywords=%28%22coronavirus%22+%22covid%22+%28coping&qid
=1586555419&sr=8-13

172. https://www.sciencemag.org/news/2020/04/
crushing-coronavirus-means-breaking-habits-lifetime-behavior-scientists-have-some-tips

173. https://pressreleases.responsesource.com/news/99708/
cuhu-launches-app-to-help-with-lockdown-mental-health-issues/

174. https://www.ncbi.nlm.nih.gov/pmc/articles/PMC3572237/

175. https://stresscenter.ucsf.edu/measures/daily-stressors

176. https://pursuit.unimelb.edu.au/articles/dealing-with-feelings-about-covid-19

177. https://healthitanalytics.com/news/
deep-learning-can-support-personalized-predictions-for-stress

<u>Emotion and personality. Vol. 1 Psychological aspect</u>[178]

<u>Emotion and personality. Vol. 2</u>[179]

<u>Emotionally aware technology could help us beat Zoom fatigue</u>[180]

<u>Employer Preparedness for Pandemic Influenza : Shifting the Conversation from Insurance to Investment</u>[181]

<u>Enforcing compliance with COVID-19 pandemic restrictions: Psychological aspects of a national security threat</u>[182]

<u>Enforcing compliance with COVID-19 pandemic restrictions: Psychological aspects of a national security threat</u>[183]

<u>Eustress</u>[184]

<u>Eustress compared with Distress</u>[185]

<u>Exercise is Essential for Well-Being During COVID-19 Pandemic</u>[186]

<u>Exercise May Protect Against Deadly COVID-19 Complication, Research Suggests</u>[187]

---

178. http://www.worldcat.org/oclc/256919626

179. http://www.worldcat.org/oclc/872314668

180. https://www.fastcompany.com/90515714/
emotionally-aware-technology-could-help-us-beat-zoom-fatigue

181. http://www.worldcat.org/oclc/810064970

182. https://www.preventionweb.net/news/view/70917

183. https://reliefweb.int/report/world/
enforcing-compliance-covid-19-pandemic-restrictions-psychological-aspects-national

184. https://en.wikipedia.org/wiki/Eustress

185. https://en.wikipedia.org/wiki/Eustress#Compared_with_distress

186. https://www.norwalkhospital.org/newsroom/article-listing/adults-exercise-and-covid19

187. https://news.virginia.edu/content/
exercise-may-protect-against-deadly-covid-19-complication-research-suggests

188. http://www.worldcat.org/oclc/1060718833

189. http://www.worldcat.org/oclc/1149142438

190. https://www.newsgram.com/childs-mental-health-covid-19-crisis/

191. https://blog.timesunion.com/capitol/archives/289763/
    free-meditation-app-for-nyers-fund-for-first-responders-cuomo/

192. https://www.ncbi.nlm.nih.gov/pmc/articles/PMC7185265/

193. https://extranet.who.int/goarn/partner-resources-content/326

194. https://thriveglobal.com/stories/halt-to-manage-emotions/

195. https://www.realsimple.com/health/preventative-health/sleep/anxiety-dreams

196. https://www.deseret.com/indepth/2020/6/13/21273906/
    coronavirus-faith-religion-health-science-link-prayer-study-longevity-covid-19-substance-use

<u>How African-Americans Can Maintain Mental, Emotional Health During Pandemic</u>[198]

<u>How Health Care Workers Can Take Care of Themselves</u>[199]

<u>How states can promote compliance with social distancing</u>[200]

<u>How stress and loneliness can make you more likely to get COVID-19</u>[201]

<u>How the brain balances feelings of stress and calm</u>[202]

<u>How to deal with anxiety caused by the coronavirus pandemic</u>[203]

<u>How To Get a Job in a Pandemic, Recession, or Economic Crisis</u>[204]

<u>A Short Guide To Get Employed FAST</u>[205]

<u>How to Practice Self-Care During the Pandemic</u>[206]

---

197. https://www.deseret.com/indepth/2020/6/13/21273906/

coronavirus-faith-religion-health-science-link-prayer-study-longevity-covid-19-substance-use

198. https://www.washingtoninformer.com/

how-african-americans-can-maintain-mental-emotional-health-during-pandemic/

199. https://hbr.org/2020/05/how-health-care-workers-can-take-care-of-themselves

200. https://hub.jhu.edu/2020/05/06/promoting-compliance-with-social-distancing/

201. http://news.rice.edu/2020/03/19/

how-stress-and-loneliness-can-make-you-more-likely-to-get-covid-19/

202. https://www.medicalnewstoday.com/articles/where-stress-lives

203. https://www.humana.com/health-and-well-being/

anxiety-about-coronavirus?cm_mmc=EmailDMT-Medicare-_-COVID19-Newsletter-_-420-_-

Hero-CovidAnxiety

204. https://www.google.com/books/edition/

How_To_Get_a_Job_in_a_Pandemic_Recession/-LLfDwAAQBAJ?hl=en&gbpv=0

205. https://www.google.com/books/edition/

How_To_Get_a_Job_in_a_Pandemic_Recession/-LLfDwAAQBAJ?hl=en&gbpv=0

206. https://www.newswise.com/coronavirus/
    how-to-practice-self-care-during-the-pandemic/?article_id=729671

207. https://www.refinery29.com/en-us/2020/03/9552059/
    things-to-do-at-home-during-coronavirus-activities

208. https://greatergood.berkeley.edu/article/item/
    how_to_support_teachers_emotional_needs_right_now

209. https://www.amazon.com/How-Survive-Pandemic-Lessons-Covid-19-ebook/dp/
    B086XC16WB/
    ref=sr_1_fkmr0_1?dchild=1&keywords=%28%22coronavirus%22+OR+%22covid%22+OR+
    %E2%80%9Ccovida%E2%80%9D%29+%28coping+OR+psychological+OR+emotional+OR
    +%22mental+health%22%29&qid=1586555237&sr=8-1-fkmr0

210. https://www.theglobeandmail.com/business/careers/management/
    article-how-to-take-advantage-of-opportunities-during-the-coronavirus-crisis/

211. https://www.verywellmind.com/how-personality-type-affects-health-4153786

212. https://journals.sagepub.com/doi/abs/10.1177/0972150914564421?journalCode=gbra

213. https://www.nationaljewish.org/health-insights/stress-and-relaxation/stress/stressors

Individual risk management strategy and potential therapeutic options for the COVID-19 pandemic[215]

Information Diet in Covid-19 Crisis; a Commentary[216]

Isolation & Depression: Strategies for Coping With the Effects of Chronic or Situational Depression Resulting from the Impact of Self Isolation: The Little Black Book of Depression[217]

It's important to protect skin[218]

Keeping a positive mindset amid COVID-19 pandemic[219]

Knowledge of COVID-19 Symptoms May Not Be Sufficient to Change Behavior[220]

Knowledge of COVID-19 Symptoms May Not Be Sufficient to Change Behavior[221]

Life Event, Stress and Illness[222]

214. http://diginole.lib.fsu.edu/islandora/object/fsu:204734/datastream/PDF/view

215. https://www.ncbi.nlm.nih.gov/pmc/articles/PMC7139252/

216. https://www.ncbi.nlm.nih.gov/pmc/articles/PMC7085861/

217. https://www.amazon.com/Isolation-Depression-Strategies-Situational-Resulting-ebook/dp/
B086WD2YP8/
ref=sr_1_3?dchild=1&keywords=%28%22coronavirus%22+%22covid%22+%28coping&qid=
1586555769&sr=8-3

218. https://www.thehindu.com/news/cities/chennai/its-important-to-protect-skin/
article31477040.ece

219. https://news.sanfordhealth.org/coronavirus-disease-2019-covid-19/coronavirus-wellness/
keeping-positive-mindset/

220. https://healthpolicy.usc.edu/evidence-base/
knowledge-of-covid-19-symptoms-may-not-be-sufficient-to-change-behavior/

221. https://healthpolicy.usc.edu/evidence-base/
knowledge-of-covid-19-symptoms-may-not-be-sufficient-to-change-behavior/

222. https://www.ncbi.nlm.nih.gov/pmc/articles/PMC3341916/

223. https://www.ptsd.va.gov/professional/assessment/te-measures/lsc-r.asp

224. https://www.forbes.com/sites/christinecomaford/2020/05/30/losing-it-so-is-everyone-else---research-provides-answers/#a5c02393e59c943d6a75a9241140faca34424b10a1246

225. https://hbr.org/2015/09/make-yourself-immune-to-secondhand-stress

226. https://www.cdc.gov/coronavirus/2019-ncov/daily-life-coping/managing-stress-anxiety.html

227. http://flcourier.com/mental-health-experts-share-ways-to-maintain-mental-emotional-health/

228. https://torontosun.com/life/relationships/0424-lifenational1

229. https://www.amazon.com/MIND-OVER-CORONAVIRUS-Win-Psychological/dp/B086L1BXDF/ref=sr_1_11?dchild=1&keywords=%28%22coronavirus%22+%22covid%22+%28coping&qid=1586555419&sr=8-11

230. https://www.sciencedirect.com/science/article/pii/S0025556420300596

My "I'm Stressed about COVID-19 and Need to Write about It" Therapeutic Journal: Journaling to Help Reduce Anxiety about the Coronavirus[232]

NC should measure children's social and emotional health, a report says. Here's how.[233]

New Device Addresses Growing Mental Health Concerns During Pandemic[234]

Nutrition amid the COVID-19 pandemic: a multi-level framework for action[235]

Nutritional recommendations for CoVID-19 quarantine[236]

Occupational stress[237]

On Coronavirus Lockdown? Look for Meaning, Not Happiness - Why cultivating "tragic optimism" will help us weather this crisis — and even grow from it.[238]

---

231. https://www.google.com/books/edition/Modeling_the_Interplay_Between_Human_Beh/
    IXhEAAAAQBAJ?hl=en&gbpv=0

232. https://www.amazon.com/Stressed-about-COVID-19-Therapeutic-Journal/dp/
    B0863TZ4KC/
    ref=sr_1_25?dchild=1&keywords=%28%22coronavirus%22+%22covid%22+%28coping&qid
    =1586555638&sr=8-25

233. https://www.ednc.org/nc-measure-young-children-social-emotional-health-ncecf-report/

234. https://menafn.com/1100343635/
    New-Device-Addresses-Growing-Mental-Health-Concerns-During-Pandemic

235. https://www.ncbi.nlm.nih.gov/pmc/articles/PMC7167535/

236. https://www.nature.com/articles/s41430-020-0635-2

237. https://en.wikipedia.org/wiki/Occupational_stress

238. https://www.nytimes.com/2020/04/07/opinion/coronavirus-mental-health.html

One in five children in China showed depressive symptoms after coronavirus quarantine. Here's how parents can help.[239]

Our Subconscious Biases Tell us Not to Social Distance[240]

Paging Dr. Within : How to Become, Be, and/or Make a "Patient Listener" and/or a "Super Symptom Checker"[241]

Pandemic Highlights Need for Measuring Kids' Social-Emotional Health[242]

Pandemic Influenza Preparedness and Response[243]

Pandemic pushing telehealth approach for physical, mental health providers[244]

Peace during uncertainty: Finding ways to maintain mental health during a pandemic[245]

Prioritizing children's freedom to play with friends to ease stress of lockdown[246]

239. https://www.inquirer.com/health/coronavirus/
coronavirus-covid19-children-mental-health-depression-20200429.html

240. https://nationalinterest.org/blog/reboot/
our-subconscious-biases-tell-us-not-social-distance-156421

241. https://books2read.com/u/mBgJnA

242. https://www.publicnewsservice.org/2020-05-21/early-childhood-education/
pandemic-highlights-need-for-measuring-kids-social-emotional-health/a70281-1

243. https://www.google.com/books/edition/Pandemic_Influenza_Preparedness_and_Resp/
vYYlWzMdHEIC?hl=en&gbpv=0

244. https://www.joplinglobe.com/coronavirus/
pandemic-pushing-telehealth-approach-for-physical-mental-health-providers/
article_52e1e487-f960-502f-9e7d-af9e7c4179c9.html

245. https://www.theunion.com/lifestyles/health/
peace-during-uncertainty-finding-ways-to-maintain-mental-health-during-a-pandemic/

Promoting Student Mental Health in Difficult Days[247]

Psychological First Aid: Guide for Field Workers[248]

Psychological stress[249]

Psychology experts share their tips for safeguarding your mental health during quarantine[250]

Reduce initial dose of the virus and optimize your immune system[251]

Reduce Stress and Anxiety Levels with Journaling - Writing about struggles and feelings may help you cope with the global pandemic.[252]

Reducing SARS-CoV-2 transmission in the UK: A behavioural science approach to identifying options for increasing adherence to social distancing and shielding vulnerable people.[253]

---

246. https://medicalxpress.com/news/2020-05-prioritizing-children-freedom-friends-ease.html

247. https://www.insidehighered.com/views/2020/05/29/

    advice-promoting-student-mental-health-during-pandemic-opinion

248. https://books.google.com/

    books?id=R3HLygAACAAJ&dq=(%22coronavirus%22+OR+%22covid%22+OR+%E2%80

    %9Ccovida%E2%80%9D)+(coping+OR+psychological+OR+emotional+OR+%22mental+h

    ealth%22)&hl=en&newbks=1&newbks_redir=0&sa=X&ved=2ahUKEwjYjfnQ7t7oAhUZO

    s0KHb0tCfI4FBDoATAEegQIAhAC

249. https://en.wikipedia.org/wiki/Psychological_stress

250. https://www.cnbc.com/2020/03/20/

    coronavirus-tips-for-protecting-your-mental-health-during-quarantine.html

251. https://peperperspective.com/2020/04/04/

    can-you-reduce-the-risk-of-coronavirus-exposure-and-optimize-your-immune-system/

252. https://www.psychologytoday.com/us/blog/evidence-based-living/202004/

    reduce-stress-and-anxiety-levels-journaling

253. http://www.worldcat.org/oclc/8596234525

Relationships Between Life Stressors, Health Behaviors, and Chronic Medical Conditions in Mid-Life Adults: A Narrative Review[254]

Saving Your Health, One Mask at a Time[255]

Sleep Guidelines During the COVID-19 Pandemic[256]

Social and environmental stressors in the home and childhood asthma[257]

Social, Cognitive, and Emotional Predictors of Adherence to Physical Distancing During the COVID-19 Pandemic[258]

Start Simple with MyPlate: Food Planning During the Coronavirus Pandemic[259]

Staying physically and mentally active during the COVID-19 lock-down[260]

Stress (biology)[261]

Stress and Health: Biological and Psychological Interactions[262]

---

254. https://www.ncbi.nlm.nih.gov/pubmed/30691935

255. https://caremesh.com/blog/2020/4/8/saving-your-health-one-mask-at-a-time

256. https://www.sleepfoundation.org/sleep-guidelines-covid-19-isolation

257. https://www.ncbi.nlm.nih.gov/pmc/articles/PMC3094102/

258. https://psyarxiv.com/ksj52/

259. https://www.choosemyplate.gov/coronavirus

260. https://pkdcharity.org.uk/news-events/blogs/
    406-staying-physically-and-mentally-active-during-the-covid-19-lock-down

261. https://en.wikipedia.org/wiki/Stress_(biology)

262. https://books.google.com/
    books?id=1KGXBgAAQBAJ&newbks=1&newbks_redir=0&dq=%22immune+system%E2%
    80%9D+(psychological+OR+emotional+OR+%22mental+health%22)&source=gbs_navlinks
    _s

263. https://www.ncbi.nlm.nih.gov/pubmed/22271841

264. http://www.worldcat.org/oclc/1048838954

265. https://thriveglobal.com/stories/
stress-symptoms-amplified-by-covid-19-leading-to-an-increase-in-teeth-grinding-although-invol
untary-there-are-steps-you-can-take-to-curb-the-impact/

266. http://pni.osumc.edu/KG%20Publications%20(pdf)/195.pdf

267. https://en.wikipedia.org/wiki/Stressor

268. http://citeseerx.ist.psu.edu/viewdoc/download?doi=10.1.1.468.8648&rep=rep1&type=pdf

269. https://www.psychologytoday.com/us/blog/hope-resilience/202004/
stressors-and-coping-mechanisms-covid-19-medical-staff

270. https://www.ncbi.nlm.nih.gov/pubmed/26032519

271. https://www.ncbi.nlm.nih.gov/pubmed/26831378

---

272. https://www.ncbi.nlm.nih.gov/pubmed/29752045

273. http://www.worldcat.org/oclc/1016946727

274. https://thehill.com/opinion/technology/
     494614-suggestions-for-telemental-health-resources-for-coping-with-covid-19

275. https://www.nimh.nih.gov/news/science-news/2020/
     supporting-mental-health-during-the-covid-19-pandemic.shtml

276. https://www.amazon.com/Coronavirus-Manual-Parents-Behavior-Claustrophobia/dp/
     1728233224

277. https://books.google.com/
     books?id=fLLWDwAAQBAJ&newbks=1&newbks_redir=0&dq=(%22coronavirus%22+OR
     +%22covid%22+OR+%E2%80%9Ccovida%E2%80%9D)+%E2%80%9Cimmune+system%E
     2%80%9D&source=gbs_navlinks_s

278. https://www.americanrivers.org/2020/03/
     the-fight-against-covid-19-must-begin-with-clean-water-for-all/

279. https://www.self.com/story/gratitude-benefits

The main articles for this category are Stress (biological) and Stress (psychological).[280]

The Persuasive Effect of Fox News : Non-Compliance with Social Distancing During the Covid-19 Pandemic[281]

The Role of Health Sciences Students During a Pandemic[282]

The Science of Helping Out - During a crisis, the people who cope best are those who help others.[283]

The surprising reasons people cheat at social distancing[284]

These Mental Habits Help Resilient People Handle Stay-at-Home Orders - It's why some people are living with the strain of social distancing better than others.[285]

Tips for tending to your mental health during the pandemic[286]

Tips to help you stay mentally healthy during the covid-19 crisis[287]

---

280. https://en.wikipedia.org/wiki/Category:Stress

281. http://www.worldcat.org/oclc/1156242231

282. https://observatory.tec.mx/edu-bits-2/the-role-of-healths-science-students-during-a-pandemic

283. https://www.nytimes.com/2020/04/09/well/mind/
coronavirus-resilience-psychology-anxiety-stress-volunteering.html

284. https://www.halifaxtoday.ca/coronavirus-covid-19-local-news/
the-surprising-reasons-people-cheat-at-social-distancing-2395432

285. https://www.inc.com/minda-zetlin/
resilient-people-mental-habits-pandemic-social-distancing-crisis.html

286. https://catholicsentinel.org/Content/News/Local/Article/
Tips-for-tending-to-your-mental-health-during-the-pandemic-/2/35/39825

287. http://www.thesuburban.com/life/lifestyles/
tips-to-help-you-stay-mentally-healthy-during-the-covid-19-crisis/
article_f51b2288-8ca3-11ea-b51d-ab9c4e7387cf.html

To manage coronavirus stress, experiment with a tried-and-true strategy - Expressive writing can benefit both physical and mental health.[288]

Today's Tip(s)[289]

Types of Stressors (Eustress vs. Distress)[290]

Using social and behavioural science to support COVID-19 pandemic response[291]

Want to Stop the COVID-19 Stress Meltdown? Train Your Brain[292]

WASH and COVID-19[293]

Water, sanitation, hygiene and waste management for COVID-19[294]

What Black mamas can do to care for their mental health[295]

What color is your parachute? : a practical manual for job-hunters and career-changers[296]

What is Stress? What is a Stressor?[297]

---

288. https://www.inverse.com/mind-body/coronavirus-stress-strategy-journaling

289. https://www.ymcafoxcities.org/sites/ymcafoxcities.org/files/2020-04/

   dailytips_week1.pdf?dxk=H4sIAAAAAAAEAKtWKs4vLUpOVbJScs1LT0xPVdJRSk7MLUj

   MTM8DimXmZZZkJpZklqUWx-gbGllamirVAgB7wrDjMwAAAA2

290. https://www.mentalhelp.net/stress/types-of-stressors-eustress-vs-distress/

291. https://www.nature.com/articles/s41562-020-0884-z

292. https://nationalinterest.org/blog/reboot/

   want-stop-covid-19-stress-meltdown-train-your-brain-162569

293. https://www.who.int/water_sanitation_health/news-events/wash-and-covid-19/en/

294. https://www.who.int/publications-detail/

   water-sanitation-hygiene-and-waste-management-for-covid-19

295. https://www.mother.ly/life/black-mothers-mental-health

296. http://www.worldcat.org/oclc/1129352773

What to Do If You Are Sick[298]

When Life Gives You a Pandemic: Stop and Smell the Flowers[299]

Who is Most Likely to Voluntarily Comply with COVID-19 Public Health Recommendations?[300]

Why children need to play with their friends as soon as they can[301]

Why it's important to get a good night's sleep during the coronavirus outbreak[302]

Why watching comedies is 'important medicine'[303]

You Are Not Alone - The stress of the pandemic can play tricks on your mind, but that doesn't mean anything is wrong with you.[304]

You can help slow the virus if you talk about it accurately online[305]

---

297. http://users.pfw.edu/young/251-Health/slides/Chapter-06.pdf

298. https://www.cdc.gov/coronavirus/2019-ncov/if-you-are-sick/steps-when-sick.html

299. https://www.amazon.com/When-Life-Gives-You-Pandemic/dp/B086B2DF5P/
   ref=sr_1_23?dchild=1&keywords=%28%22coronavirus%22+%22covid%22+%28coping&qid
   =1586555638&sr=8-23

300. https://www.boisestate.edu/bluereview/
   who-is-most-likely-to-voluntarily-comply-with-covid-19-public-health-recommendations/

301. https://www.thejakartapost.com/life/2020/05/18/
   why-children-need-to-play-with-their-friends-as-soon-as-they-can.html

302. https://www.uchicagomedicine.org/forefront/coronavirus-disease-covid-19/
   advice-for-sleeping-well-during-the-covid-19-outbreak

303. https://www.cbc.ca/comedy/why-watching-comedies-is-important-medicine-1.5519839

304. https://washingtonmonthly.com/2020/04/27/its-okay-to-panic/

305. https://www.washingtonpost.com/outlook/2020/04/28/
   you-can-help-slow-virus-if-you-talk-about-it-accurately-online/

Drug use to cope with emotions or boredom can worsen physical, mental health: Health Ministry[306]

Support platform for emotional health before COVID-19[307]

JUMP BACK TO Chapter 4 – Coronavirus Treatment Information

****

REFERENCES for Chapter 4 – Coronavirus Treatment Information

'Faster protection with less material'[308] – How a new vaccine adjuvant might eventually help to shorten the race to COVID-19 immunity

A Cure Within: Scientists Unleashing the Immune System to Kill Cancer[309]

A doctor's reassurance speeds healing from an allergic reaction, find Stanford psychologists[310]

---

306. https://www.thehindu.com/news/national/
    drug-use-to-cope-with-emotions-or-boredom-can-worsen-physical-mental-health-health-ministr
    y/article31883232.ece

307. https://www.explica.co/support-platform-for-emotional-health-before-covid-19/

308. https://news.harvard.edu/gazette/story/2020/04/
    how-a-new-vaccine-adjuvant-might-shorten-race-to-covid-19-immunity/

309. https://books.google.com/
    books?id=0BJHMQAACAAJ&dq=(%22coronavirus%22+OR+%22covid%22+OR+%E2%8
    0%9Ccovida%E2%80%9D)+%E2%80%9Cimmune+system%E2%80%9D&hl=en&newbks=1
    &newbks_redir=0&sa=X&ved=2ahUKEwjGht_X897oAhXHZs0KHSI4Dt84KBDoATAGe
    gQIABAC

310. https://news.stanford.edu/2018/09/04/doctors-reassurance-speeds-healing/

A new clinical trial to test high-dose vitamin C in patients with COVID-19[311]

A placebo can work even when you know it's a placebo[312]

A review of the effects of hypnosis on the immune system in breast cancer patients: a brief communication.[313]

Adjuvant[314]

Adjuvants for pandemic influenza vaccines.[315]

Adjuvants: vaccines' hidden helpers[316]

As coronavirus fears mount, some seek alternative healing[317]

Ayurveda and COVID-19: where psychoneuroimmunology and the meaning response meet[318]

Ayurveda and COVID-19: Where psychoneuroimmunology and the meaning response meet[319]

Call to Action: Announcing the Traditional, Complementary and Integrative Health and Medicine COVID-19 Support Registry[320]

---

311. https://www.ncbi.nlm.nih.gov/pmc/articles/PMC7137406/

312. https://www.health.harvard.edu/blog/placebo-can-work-even-know-placebo-201607079926

313. https://www.ncbi.nlm.nih.gov/pubmed/17786658

314. https://en.wikipedia.org/wiki/Adjuvant

315. https://www.ncbi.nlm.nih.gov/pubmed/19768413

316. https://www.chemistryworld.com/features/adjuvants-vaccines-hidden-helpers/4011156.article

317. https://www.jpost.com/HEALTH-SCIENCE/
     As-coronavirus-fears-mount-some-seek-alternative-healing-625010

318. https://www.ncbi.nlm.nih.gov/pmc/articles/PMC7175849/

319. https://www.ncbi.nlm.nih.gov/pmc/articles/PMC7175849/

320. https://pubmed.ncbi.nlm.nih.gov/32250655/

Can Hypnosis or Hypnotherapy Help Strengthen the Immune System?[321]

Chronic stress alters the immune response to influenza virus vaccine in older adults[322]

Cold Vaccines - An Evaluation Based On A Controlled Study[323]

COVID-19 and vitamin D—Is there a link and an opportunity for intervention?[324]

COVID-19: Melatonin as a potential adjuvant treatment[325]

CURED : the life-changing science of spontaneous healing.[326]

Designing a coronavirus vaccine for next year – and the years beyond[327]

Do placebos have a place in clinical practice?[328]

Do placebos provide a mental cue to kickstart the immune system?[329]

Effects of acute psychological stress on placebo and nocebo responses in a clinically relevant model of visceroception[330]

321. https://web.wellness-institute.org/blog/bid/399304/
Can-Hypnosis-or-Hypnotherapy-Help-Strengthen-the-Immune-System

322. https://www.ncbi.nlm.nih.gov/pmc/articles/PMC39758/

323. https://jamanetwork.com/journals/jama/article-abstract/282478

324. https://journals.physiology.org/doi/full/10.1152/ajpendo.00138.2020

325. https://www.ncbi.nlm.nih.gov/pmc/articles/PMC7102583/

326. http://www.worldcat.org/oclc/1079847198

327. https://discoveries.childrenshospital.org/coronavirus-vaccine/

328. https://acpinternist.org/archives/2009/04/placebo.htm

329. https://scopeblog.stanford.edu/2012/09/06/
do-placebos-provide-a-mental-cue-to-kickstart-the-immune-system/

330. https://journals.lww.com/pain/Abstract/2017/08000/
Effects_of_acute_psychological_stress_on_placebo.13.aspx

Efficacy of Natural Honey Treatment in Patients With Novel Coronavirus[331]

Got Coronavirus Antibodies?[332]

Harnessing the Placebo Effect: Exploring the Influenceof Physician Characteristics on Placebo Response[333]

High-Dose IV Vitamin C on ARDS by COVID-19: A Possible Low-Cost Ally With a Wide Margin of Safety[334]

How a doctor's words can make you ill[335]

How the doctor's words affect the patient's brain.[336]

How to Maximize Motivation in a Patient[337]

How to Personalize the Placebo Effect, similar to Personalized Medicine[338]

Human Psychoneuroimmunology[339]

Hypnobo: Perspectives on Hypnosis and Placebo[340]

331. https://clinicaltrials.gov/ct2/show/NCT04323345

332. https://www.wsj.com/articles/got-coronavirus-antibodies-11585782003

333. https://mbl.stanford.edu/sites/g/files/sbiybj9941/f/
howegoyercrum_harnessingtheplaceboeffect.pdf

334. https://www.physiciansweekly.com/
high-dose-iv-vitamin-c-on-ards-by-covid-19-a-possible-low-cost-ally-with-a-wide-margin-of-safety/

335. https://www.bbc.com/future/article/20150309-the-simple-words-that-make-us-ill

336. https://www.ncbi.nlm.nih.gov/pubmed/12449081

337. https://interesting-health-information.blogspot.com/2018/08/
how-to-maximize-motivation-in-patient.html

338. https://tgideas.blogspot.com/2018/11/how-to-personalize-placebo-effect.html

339. https://books.google.com/
    books?id=zPy6Y1fZy8QC&newbks=1&newbks_redir=0&dq=%22immune+system%E2%80
    %9D+(psychological+OR+emotional+OR+%22mental+health%22)&source=gbs_navlinks_s

340. https://razlab.mcgill.ca/docs/Hypnobo.pdf

341. https://news.osu.edu/hypnosis-may-prevent-weakened-immune-status-improve-health/

342. https://www.ncbi.nlm.nih.gov/pmc/articles/PMC3312698/

343. https://en.wikipedia.org/wiki/Immunologic_adjuvant

344. https://books.google.com/
    books?id=cWJ7DwAAQBAJ&newbks=1&newbks_redir=0&dq=%22immune+system%E2%
    80%9D+(psychological+OR+emotional+OR+%22mental+health%22)&source=gbs_navlinks
    _s

345. https://en.wikipedia.org/wiki/Immunostimulant

346. https://academic.oup.com/jnci/article/95/1/6/2520179

347. https://www.kpbs.org/news/2016/oct/27/is-it-still-a-placebo-when-it-works-and-you-know/

348. https://www.ncbi.nlm.nih.gov/pmc/articles/PMC2928990/

349. https://en.wikipedia.org/wiki/List_of_unproven_methods_against_COVID-19

---

350. http://interesting-health-information.blogspot.com/search/label/spontaneous%20healing

351. http://www.worldcat.org/oclc/940658166

352. https://otd.harvard.edu/explore-innovation/technologies/
    novel-adjuvants-to-enhance-adaptive-immune-response-of-vaccines

353. https://www.ncbi.nlm.nih.gov/pmc/articles/PMC1114024/

354. https://clinicaltrials.gov/ct2/show/NCT04366089

355. https://books2read.com/u/mBgJnA

356. https://www.psychologytoday.com/us/blog/the-new-normal/202004/
    pandemics-and-psychoneuroimmunology

357. https://time.com/5375724/placebo-bill-health-problems/

358. https://www.washingtonpost.com/news/health-science/wp/2016/12/02/
    people-susceptible-to-the-placebo-effect-may-be-keeping-us-from-getting-new-drugs/

Personality Predicts Placebo Effect[359]

Personalized treatment management system[360]

Person-centered osteopathic practice: patients' personality (body, mind, and soul) and health (ill-being and well-being)[361]

Placebo[362]

Placebo - The Power of Words[363]

Placebo and Belief Effects: Optimal Design for Randomized Trials[364]

Placebo and the New Physiology of the Doctor-Patient Relationship[365]

Placebo effect may reveal some of its secrets in new study[366]

Placebo Effects and the Common Cold: A Randomized Controlled Trial[367]

Placebo effects in allergen immunotherapy: an experts' opinion[368]

Placebo Effects in the Immune System.[369]

---

359. https://www.the-scientist.com/daily-news/personality-predicts-placebo-effect-40178

360. http://appft1.uspto.gov/netacgi/
nph-Parser?Sect1=PTO1&Sect2=HITOFF&d=PG01&p=1&u=/netahtml/PTO/
srchnum.html&r=1&f=G&l=50&s1=20180089385

361. https://www.ncbi.nlm.nih.gov/pubmed/26528411

362. https://en.wikipedia.org/wiki/Placebo

363. https://scholarworks.umt.edu/cgi/viewcontent.cgi?article=2747&context=syllabi

364. http://faculty.wcas.northwestern.edu/~sro850/BeliefEffects.pdf

365. https://www.ncbi.nlm.nih.gov/pmc/articles/PMC3962549/

366. https://www.statnews.com/2016/07/04/placebo-effect-brain-immune-system/

367. https://www.ncbi.nlm.nih.gov/pmc/articles/PMC3133578/

368. https://www.ncbi.nlm.nih.gov/pmc/articles/PMC6132371/

369. https://www.ncbi.nlm.nih.gov/pubmed/29681334

Placebo Effects on the Immune Response in Humans: The Role of Learning and Expectation[370]

Placebo Improves Asthma Symptoms, But Not Lung Function[371]

Placebo interventions, placebo effects and clinical practice[372]

Placebos and placebo effects in medicine: historical overview[373]

Placebos by prescription may work like medicine[374]

Placebos in Medicine: Knowledge, Beliefs, and Patterns of Use[375]

Positive Thinking, Faster Recovery[376]

Practising evidence-based medicine in an era of high placebo response: number needed to treat reconsidered[377]

Prescribing Hope: The Placebo Effect Endures[378]

Prescribing Placebos[379]

Program in Placebo Studies & Therapeutic Encounter (PiPS)[380]

370. https://www.ncbi.nlm.nih.gov/pmc/articles/PMC3504052/

371. https://www.nih.gov/news-events/nih-research-matters/
     placebo-improves-asthma-symptoms-not-lung-function

372. https://www.ncbi.nlm.nih.gov/pmc/articles/PMC3130396/

373. https://www.ncbi.nlm.nih.gov/pmc/articles/PMC1297390/pdf/jrsocmed00004-0023.pdf

374. https://www.israel21c.org/placebos-by-prescription-may-work-like-medicine/

375. https://www.ncbi.nlm.nih.gov/pmc/articles/PMC2582662/

376. https://abcnews.go.com/Health/story?id=117317&page=1

377. https://www.ncbi.nlm.nih.gov/pmc/articles/PMC4853640/

378. https://www.the-rheumatologist.org/article/
     prescribing-hope-the-placebo-effect-endures/?singlepage=1&theme=print-friendly&fbclid=Iw
     AR0rh4j1PvZnjorsbutpmmgrtZLEwcFCfbbvt-ldPBcFIIsHGjui-G896I4

379. https://journalofethics.ama-assn.org/article/prescribing-placebos/2006-06

Psychological Changes Preceding Spontaneous Remission of Cancer[381]

Psychoneuroimmunology[382]

Psychoneuroimmunology : stress, mental disorders, and health[383]

Psychoneuroimmunology : Volume 2 and 1.[384]

Psychoneuroimmunology Research Society[385]

Psychoneuroimmunology: a holistic framework for the study of stress and illness[386]

Psychoneuroimmunology: An Interdisciplinary Introduction[387]

Psychoneuroimmunology: laugh and be well[388]

Psychoneuroimmunology: stress effects on pathogenesis and immunity during infection.[389]

Psychoneuroimmunology: the biological basis of the placebo phenomenon?[390]

380. http://programinplacebostudies.org/

381. http://citeseerx.ist.psu.edu/viewdoc/download?doi=10.1.1.872.7236&rep=rep1&type=pdf

382. https://en.wikipedia.org/wiki/Psychoneuroimmunology

383. http://www.worldcat.org/oclc/784301099

384. http://www.worldcat.org/oclc/814468065

385. https://www.pnirs.org/

386. https://www.ncbi.nlm.nih.gov/pubmed/2061356

387. https://books.google.com/
    books?id=ghkkKrZTOqIC&newbks=1&newbks_redir=0&dq=%22immune+system%E2%80
    %9D+(psychological+OR+emotional+OR+%22mental+health%22)&source=gbs_navlinks_s

388. https://www.medicalnewstoday.com/articles/305921

389. https://www.ncbi.nlm.nih.gov/pmc/articles/PMC358318/

390. https://www.ncbi.nlm.nih.gov/pubmed/9127260

Psychoneuroimmunology:Psychological Influences on Immune Function and Health[391]

Psychosomatic medicine[392]

Publications on the use of TCM to treat COVID-19[393]

Ritual in Western Medicine and Its Role in Placebo Healing[394]

Society for Interdisciplinary Placebo Studies (SIPS)[395]

Spontaneous Healing[396]

Spontaneous regression : cancer and the immune system[397]

Spontaneous remission[398]

Spontaneous remission : an annotated bibliography[399]

Spontaneous Remission Bibliography Project[400]

Spontaneous Remission of Cancer: Theories from Healers, Physicians, and Cancer Survivors[401]

---

391. http://citeseerx.ist.psu.edu/viewdoc/download?doi=10.1.1.521.4556&rep=rep1&type=pdf

392. https://en.wikipedia.org/wiki/Psychosomatic_medicine

393. https://exploreim.ucla.edu/covid19/
publications-on-traditional-chinese-medicine-tcm-to-treat-covid-19/

394. https://profiles.wustl.edu/en/publications/
ritual-in-western-medicine-and-its-role-in-placebo-healing

395. https://www.placebosociety.org/

396. http://www.worldcat.org/oclc/843015059

397. http://www.worldcat.org/oclc/60349328

398. https://en.wikipedia.org/wiki/Spontaneous_remission

399. http://www.worldcat.org/oclc/606498894

400. https://noetic.org/research/spontaneous-remission-bibliography-project/

401. http://escholarship.ucop.edu/uc/item/3px3w4g9

Stress management and psychoneuroimmunology in HIV infection.[402]

Psychoneuroimmunology: Topics by Science.gov[403]

The brouhaha around placebo choice in vaccine trials[404]

The Connection Between Spontaneous Remission of Cancer and MindBody Medicine[405]

The nocebo effect of drugs[406]

THE PANDEMIC VACCINE PUZZLE Part 4: The promise and problems of adjuvants[407]

The Placebo Effect Is Real. Now Doctors Just Have To Work Out How To Use It[408]

The Placebo Effect: Cough and Other Conditions It Improves[409]

The Placebo Effect: Usage, Mechanisms, and Legality[410]

The placebo response in clinical trials: more questions than answers[411]

402. https://www.ncbi.nlm.nih.gov/pubmed/12627048

403. https://www.science.gov/topicpages/p/psychoneuroimmunology.html

404. https://sciblogs.co.nz/diplomaticimmunity/2018/02/21/
the-brouhaha-around-placebo-choice-in-vaccine-trials/

405. https://pdfs.semanticscholar.org/c3d8/f4dd388669269528c299f433e71018be23c4.pdf

406. https://www.ncbi.nlm.nih.gov/pmc/articles/PMC4804316/

407. https://www.cidrap.umn.edu/news-perspective/2007/10/
pandemic-vaccine-puzzle-part-4-promise-and-problems-adjuvants

408. https://www.fastcompany.com/3016012/
the-placebo-effect-is-real-now-doctors-just-have-to-work-out-how-to-use-it

409. https://abcnews.go.com/Health/placebo-effect-coughs-conditions-improves/
story?id=16612769

410. https://www.uspharmacist.com/article/the-placebo-effect-usage-mechanisms-and-legality

411. https://www.ncbi.nlm.nih.gov/pmc/articles/PMC3130397/

The placebo response: how words and rituals change the patient's brain.[412]

The Radical Remission Project[413]

The Role of Patient–Practitioner Relationships in Placebo and Nocebo Phenomena[414]

The role of placebo effects in immune-related conditions: mechanisms and clinical considerations.[415]

The Use of Adjuvant Therapy in Preventing Progression to Severe Pneumonia in Patients with Coronavirus Disease 2019: A Multicenter Data Analysis[416]

The Vaccination Model in Psychoneuroimmunology Research: A Review[417]

The Wiley-Blackwell Handbook of Psychoneuroimmunology[418]

The Will to Live[419]

---

412. https://www.ncbi.nlm.nih.gov/pubmed/21621366

413. https://radicalremission.com/

414. https://www.ncbi.nlm.nih.gov/pmc/articles/PMC6176716/

415. https://www.ncbi.nlm.nih.gov/pubmed/30139289

416. https://www.medrxiv.org/content/10.1101/2020.04.08.20057539v1

417. https://pubmed.ncbi.nlm.nih.gov/
29705854/?fbclid=IwAR3DEyofnuP_CTf0-oTuVL117D87Fn-vO2lAPqhtvVuNs3VdJLsoa2qk
VAA

418. https://books.google.com/
books?id=zzdtDwAAQBAJ&newbks=1&newbks_redir=0&dq=%22immune+system%E2%8
0%9D+(psychological+OR+emotional+OR+%22mental+health%22)&source=gbs_navlinks_
s

419. https://psychcentral.com/lib/the-will-to-live/

These Fake Pills May Help You Feel Better[420]

Twenty years of psychoneuroimmunology and viral infections in Brain, Behavior, and Immunity.[421]

Two known therapies could be useful as adjuvant therapy in critical patients infected by COVID-19.[422]

Understanding the placebo effect in complementary medicine : theory, practice and research[423]

Use of Saline as a Placebo in Intra-articular Injections in Osteoarthritis: Potential Contributions to Nociceptive Pain Relief[424]

Using "Number Needed to Treat" to Interpret Treatment Effect[425]

Using psychoneuroimmunity against COVID-19[426]

Vaccination and the placebo effect[427]

Vaccine[428]

Vitamin D on Prevention and Treatment of COVID-19 (COVITD-19)[429]

Vitamins as influenza vaccine adjuvant components.[430]

420. https://www.sciencemag.org/news/2010/12/these-fake-pills-may-help-you-feel-better

421. https://www.ncbi.nlm.nih.gov/pubmed/17158025

422. https://www.ncbi.nlm.nih.gov/pubmed/32303365

423. http://www.worldcat.org/oclc/248234306

424. https://www.ncbi.nlm.nih.gov/pmc/articles/PMC5366377/

425. http://www.ant-tnsjournal.com/Mag_Files/15-2/15-2_p120.pdf

426. https://www.ncbi.nlm.nih.gov/pubmed/32234338

427. https://www.thelancet.com/journals/laninf/article/PIIS1473-3099(06)70503-5/fulltext

428. https://en.wikipedia.org/wiki/Vaccine

429. https://clinicaltrials.gov/ct2/show/NCT04334005

What Is an Adjuvant, and Why Are They Used in Vaccines?[431]

What is the Placebo Effect?[432]

When and Why Placebo-Prescribing Is Acceptable and Unacceptable: A Focus Group Study of Patients' Views[433]

Will to live[434]

JUMP BACK TO Chapter 5 – Conclusion

****

GOOD SEARCH STRINGS... related to this book...to "Find More Like This"...

How to Find Anything Online With Advanced Search Techniques[435]

Google Guide Cheat Sheet[436]

"immune system" (strong OR strengthen OR boost OR enhance OR augment OR improve)

("coronavirus" OR "covid" OR "covida") (placebo OR hypnosis OR hypnotherapy OR "guided imagery")

---

430. https://www.ncbi.nlm.nih.gov/pubmed/27449155

431. https://www.chop.edu/centers-programs/vaccine-education-center/video/
    what-adjuvant-and-why-are-they-used-vaccines

432. https://www.drugs.com/article/placebo-effect.html

433. https://www.ncbi.nlm.nih.gov/pmc/articles/PMC4089920/

434. https://en.wikipedia.org/wiki/Will_to_live

435. https://computers.tutsplus.com/tutorials/
    how-to-find-anything-online-with-advanced-search-techniques--cms-21154

436. http://www.googleguide.com/print/adv_op_ref.pdf

("coronavirus" OR "covid" OR "covida") (psychological OR emotional OR "mental health")

("coronavirus" OR "covid" OR "covida") "diet"

("coronavirus" OR "covid" OR "covida") "immune system"

("coronavirus" OR "covid" OR virus OR viral) "stressor"

("coronavirus" OR "covid") "immune system" (strong OR strengthen OR boost OR enhance OR augment OR improve)

("coronavirus" OR "covid") ("new normal" OR "after effects")

("coronavirus" OR "covid") (natural OR herd) immunity

("coronavirus" OR "covid") (stress OR stressor OR depression)

("immune system" OR "immunity") (placebo OR hypnosis OR hypnotherapy OR "guided imagery")

("immune system" OR "immunity") (placebo OR hypnosis OR hypnotherapy OR "guided imagery")

("immune system" OR immunity) (strong OR strengthen OR boost OR enhance OR augment OR improve) (placebo OR hypnosis OR hypnotherapy OR "guided imagery")

("immune system" OR immunity) "placebo"

("immune system" OR immunity) "placebo" (needles OR injection OR hypodermic OR shot)

("immune system") (psychological OR emotional OR "mental health")

("stressor" OR "stress" OR "distress") "vaccine" (effectiveness)

(coronavirus OR covid OR covida)

(coronavirus OR covid) "immune system"

(psychoneuroimmunology OR (PNI) OR psychoendoneuroimmunology OR (PENI) OR psychoneuroendocrinoimmunology OR (PNEI)) ("coronavirus" OR "covid")

(psychoneuroimmunology OR (PNI) OR psychoendoneuroimmunology OR (PENI) OR psychoneuroendocrinoimmunology OR (PNEI) OR "immune system" OR immunity) "placebo"

(psychoneuroimmunology OR (PNI) OR psychoendoneuroimmunology OR (PENI) OR psychoneuroendocrinoimmunology OR (PNEI) OR "immune system" OR immunity) ("hypnosis" OR "hypnotherapy")

(psychoneuroimmunology OR (PNI) OR psychoendoneuroimmunology OR (PENI) OR psychoneuroendocrinoimmunology OR (PNEI)) ("immune system" OR immunity) (strong OR strengthen OR boost OR enhance OR augment OR improve) (placebo OR hypnosis OR hypnotherapy OR "guided imagery")

"placebo" ("coronavirus" OR "covid" OR virus OR viral)

"placebo" (ritual OR words OR actions) ("doctor" OR "physician")

JUMP BACK TO APPENDIX

****

Contact me –

Tom Garz - TG Ideas LLC[437]

---

437. https://sites.google.com/site/tgideas/

691 S. Green Bay Rd. # 180

Neenah, WI 54956 U.S.A.

E-Mail tgideas@gmail.com

JUMP BACK TO APPENDIX

Don't miss out!

Visit the website below and you can sign up to receive emails whenever Tom Garz publishes a new book. There's no charge and no obligation.

https://books2read.com/r/B-A-BDUH-QTUGB

BOOKS 2 READ

Connecting independent readers to independent writers.

Also by Tom Garz

Paging Dr. Within: How to Become, Be, and/or Make a "Patient Listener" and/or a "Super Symptom Checker"
Coronavirus-The Inside Story: Multidimensional Prevention and Treatment
Living Through This Pandemic: "Just for Today"
Over 700 Ways to Live "Just for Today"

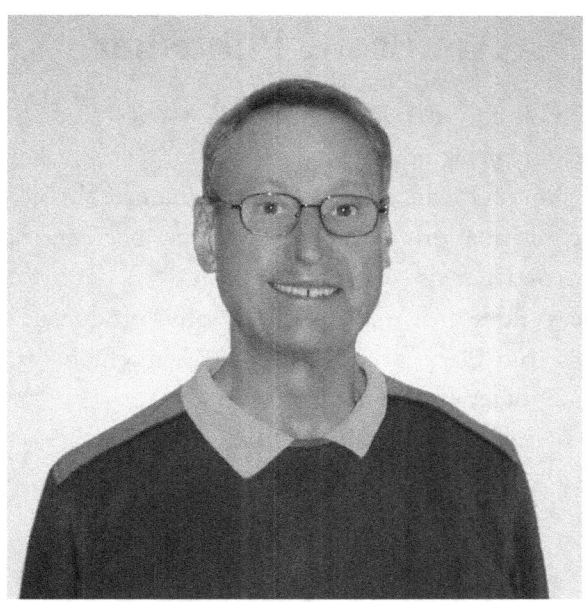

About the Author

Tom Garz is the manager of TG Ideas LLC - writing and inventing, since 2003.

"Helping to make this a better world by providing information to others on what has been done already and offer up ideas on what else might be done"

Tom has a technical background, a B.S. in Physics, and has worked in variety of jobs in his life. He always has had an interest in Electronics and "fringe science". "Exploring" is one of his favorite activities. Tom has a keen interest in writing and inventing.

Tom hopes you find his books beneficial for you and/or others. :-)

Tom might be available as a Consultant. Contact TG Ideas LLC, if interested.

tgideas@gmail.com

About the Publisher

TG Ideas LLC is a limited liability company registered in Wisconsin. It was formed in Spring of 2003.

The Mission of TG Ideas LLC is to "Help make this a better world by providing information to others on what has been done already and offer up ideas on what else might be done"

TG Ideas does not make or sell any products, other than publications. Tom Garz, of TG Ideas LLC, might be available as a Consultant. Contact - tgideas@gmail.com

https://sites.google.com/site/tgideas/